The Feeling Child: Affective Development Reconsidered

The *Journal of Children in Contemporary Society* series:

- *Young Children in a Computerized Environment*
- *Primary Prevention for Children & Families*
- *The Puzzling Child: From Recognition to Treatment*
- *Children of Exceptional Parents*
- *Childhood Depression*
- *Newcomers to the United States: Children and Families*
- *Child Care: Emerging Legal Issues*
- *A Child's Brain: The Impact of Advanced Research on Cognitive and Social Behaviors*
- *Teachers: Economic Growth and Society*
- *Infant Intervention Programs: Truths and Untruths*
- *Marketing Child Care Programs: Why and How*
- *Competent Caregivers—Competent Children: Training and Education for Child Care Practice*
- *The Feeling Child: Affective Development Reconsidered*

The Feeling Child: Affective Development Reconsidered

Edited by
Nancy E. Curry, PhD

The Haworth Press
New York • London

The Feeling Child: Affective Development Reconsidered has also been published as *Journal of Children in Contemporary Society,* Volume 17, Number 4, Summer 1985.

The Haworth Press, Inc., 28 East 22 Street, New York, NY 10010-6194
EUROSPAN/Haworth, 3 Henrietta Street, London WC2E 8LU England

Library of Congress Cataloging-in-Publication Data

The Feeling child.

"Has also been published as Journal of children in contemporary society, volume 17, number 4, summer 1985"—T.p. verso.
Bibliography: p.
Includes index.
1. Emotions in children—Addresses, essays, lectures. 2. Child development—Addresses, essays, lectures. I. Curry, Nancy E.
BF723.E6F44 1986 155.4'12 86-3068
ISBN 0-86656-555-8

The Feeling Child: Affective Development Reconsidered

Journal of Children in Contemporary Society
Volume 17, Number 4

CONTENTS

CLINICAL CONTRIBUTIONS

SELECTED READINGS

About the Editor

Nancy E. Curry, Ph.D., is Professor and Program Director, Program in Child Development and Child Care in the School of Health Related Professions, University of Pittsburgh. One of her major research interests concerns the sociodramatic play of young children with its implication for curricular and therapeutic uses; she has published a number of articles on play. In 1972 she conducted a major conference on play in conjunction with the National Association of Young Children entitled *Play: The Child Strives Toward Self-Realization.* From this conference came a NAEYC monograph by the same title. As associate director of a film project funded by the U.S. Office of Education, Dr. Curry, along with the project director Dr. Sara Arnaud, has developed 12 films depicting the developmental and cultural aspects of children's play. The major films of these series are *Role Enactment in Children's Play: A Developmental Overview, The Facilitation of Children's Play,* and *Play and Cultural Continuity, Part I-IV.* She was the former associate director of the Arsenal Family & Children's Center. In addition to her teaching at the University of Pittsburgh, Dr. Curry has been a visiting professor at Oregon State University and Arizona State University. She spent a year in England as a Fulbright Exchange teacher at the North Oxford Nursery School. Her national consultantships have included the Bureau of Indian Affairs, Operation Headstart, Allyn & Bacon Publishing Company and Child Development Group of Mississippi. In Pittsburgh, she is a consultant to the St. Andrew's Nursery School, Parents' United, Pittsburgh First-Born Project and Pittsburgh Catholic Head Start. Currently, she is a research associate of the Pittsburgh Psychoanalytic Institute.

Preface

In today's highly technological and mechanized society with a heavy emphasis on the importance of cognitive skills and strategies, there seems to be a concomitant lack of attention to the emotional life of children. We are once again experiencing the pendulum swing between the cognitive and affective approaches to dealing with children both educationally and therapeutically. Although this dichotomy has been addressed frequently over the years, it seems timely to acknowledge and to explore the highly sophisticated body of theoretical and applied knowledge that is accruing concerning the importance of affective development. This issue is an attempt to collate that knowledge, to offer support to those who are committed to affective education and treatment programs, to update the recent research findings in affective development, and to open new avenues for research, educational planning and therapeutic planning in the field of affective development. In today's complicated world, children are confronted with challenges which cognitive strategies are being developed. How children feel about these challenges and how their feelings color the way they approach problems needs to be addressed and understood.

Psychoanalysis, with its rich history of exploring the affects and their vicissitudes, has provided the most extensive body of knowledge covering affective development. The earliest and the most recent psychoanalytic writers, however, have acknowledged that it is difficult to develop a unified theory of affects. With new methods of observation and with the closer attention given to the development of infants, we are witnessing a groundswell of research interest on the part of psychologists, as well as psychoanalysts, in the area of affective development. Many clinicians and educators have continued a steady exploration of the importance of affects in their writings and in direct work, but this exploration tends to be imbedded in a variety of other subject areas and thus, often scattered throughout the literature.

This issue, then, focuses on the recent developments in the area of affective development in terms of theory, research and practice from the theoretical perspectives of psychoanalysis, social psychology, developmental psychology, family therapy and child development. Further, the affective development of children with both physical and social handicapping conditions and those coping with environmental stresses and stimulation is considered. This volume contains valuable insights from such eminent theoreticians and clinicians as Stanley Greenspan, M.D., Michael Lewis, Ph.D., Maria Piers, Ph.D. and Sally Provence, M.D. Their contributions are buttressed and extended by the research findings of Gilbert Foley, Ed.D., Dorothy Singer, Ph.D., Jerome Singer, Ph.D., and Janet Strayer, Ph.D. For practical guidance to educators, clinicians and others who work with young children, the clinical contributions of Nancy E. Curry, Ph.D., Victoria Dimidjian, Ph.D. and Hugh Crago, M.Litt., M.A. give careful consideration to the ways children's affective lives can be ameliorated and enhanced. The guest editor wishes to acknowledge these authors for the careful thought and hard work that went into each of these contributions, as well as Mary Frank, M.Ed., editor of the *Journal of Children in Contemporary Society*.

Nancy E. Curry
Guest Editor

Introduction

Stanley Greenspan, MD

Understanding the nature and processes of normal child development, and especially the development of those qualities that are distinctly human, has been a challenge since early times. The current "nature versus nurture" debates interestingly reflect many of the same basic questions that were addressed in the past. The debates have included questions of the degree to which developmental potentials and patterns are already present at conception, the effect of the environment on modifying those potentials and patterns, and, at the other extreme, the degree to which environmental experiences fill in the relatively "blank tablet" of human potentials.

Current views of development are, for the most part, balanced; they respect both genetic endowment and environmental experience, as well as the organism's capacity to structure and restructure experience—biological and environmental—at each stage of development in accordance with maturational capacities and adaptive goals.

Personality develops along multiple lines. Development in the overall physical, neurological, cognitive, and intellectual realm, as well as the development of human relationships, coping strategies, and general styles of organizing and differentiating thoughts, wishes, and feelings, contributes to the ways one organizes and creates one's unique experience of life. In addition, every discrete behavior is multiply determined. For example, a boy may be angry one day because a friend took his favorite game. He may be angry on another day because a girl flirted with him, and he became sexually aroused. He may become angry at another time because he cannot understand the teacher's math instructions. On still

Stanley I. Greenspan, Chief, Clinical Infant-Child Development Research Center, DMCH-HRSA and NIMH, 11710 Hunters Lane, Rockville, MD 20852.

another day, he may be angry because his visiting grandparents have now gone home. On yet another day, he may be angry for all those reasons at the same time.

As one considers the multiple determinants of behavior and the multiple lines of development, it becomes increasingly necessary to have a model or a way of viewing development that is sensitive to emotional functioning and that is useful to clinicians in their tasks of direct observation of children's experience. A model we have developed is the developmental-structuralist approach (Greenspan, 1979, 1981, 1985). It focuses on how a person organizes experience at each stage of development. Experience is broadly defined to encompass emotional experience, as well as experience with the inanimate or impersonal world. The person's experiential organization is the final common pathway for multiple determinants—environmental, biological, and so on—that influence behavior and can be studied in relation to each specific line of development.

Two assumptions are related to this approach. One is that a person's organizational capacity progresses to higher levels as that person matures. Higher levels, in this context, imply an ability to organize an increasingly wide and complex range of experience into stable patterns. The interplay between age-appropriate experience and maturation of the CNS ultimately determines the characteristics of this organizational capacity at each phase. The second assumption is that, for each phase of development, in addition to a characteristic organizational level, there are also certain characteristic types of experience—for example, interests or inclinations—that "play themselves out" within the organizational structure. Stage-specific experiences or inclinations are evidenced in the stage-specific types of wishes, fears, curiosities, and inclinations, which are often referred to as drives or psychosocial tasks. The model being described here is a biological adaptational one, in that the adapting person develops unique experiential organizations and contents from an interplay in which maturational progression and it's phase-specific inclinations operate on and are responded to by the environment. Stage-specific experiences are also related to the interplay between biological maturational processes and ongoing experience with the environment.

One may, therefore, usefully focus on two components of a person's experiential world. One component is the level of organization of experience. For example, one expects an 8-year-old girl to organize her experience sufficiently to be able to separate reality from fantasy, modulate impulses, regulate mood, focus her concentration, integrate thoughts and emotions, delineate—in an ever-subtler fashion—her sense of self from her sense of others, and maintain her self-esteem. The above abilities are the age-appropriate organizational features that characterize the adaptive experiential organization of an 8 year-old. In contrast, a maladaptive organization is characterized by the tendency toward disorganization, with vulnerable reality testing or impulse regulation.

The second component of a person's experiential world relates to the type of experience organized. Here, one looks at the specific thoughts, concerns, inclinations, wishes, and fears.

Categories of experience found to be clinically useful in observing the range of human endeavors that a child is able to engage in include: (1) interest and attentiveness; (2) relaxation or calmness or both; (3) dependency, including holding or comforting types of behavior; (4) pleasure or joy, including enthusiasm; (5) assertiveness—explorativeness and curiosity; (6) protest or other distinct forms of unpleasure, including anger; (7) negativism or stubbornness; (8) self-limit setting, often not seen until children are in the middle of the second year of life; and (9) after the age of 3 years, empathy and more stable feelings of love.

Each of these experiential domains may have many distinct contents. One 2-1/2-year-old boy expresses assertiveness or anger by shooting guns, another boy by beating up his father, and another child by winning a car race. Similarly, pleasure may be reflected in the excitement of feeding and undressing dolls or in the joy of building a huge tower. The contributions of psychoanalytic observers and psychosexual theory toward understanding the phase-specific organizing fantasies or dramas are of inestimable importance in the study of what contributes to distinctly human experience.

It is interesting to note that, although in the first or second month it is difficult to observe all these affective-thematic areas, by 4 months of age, it is possible to clinically observe each of these affective-thematic areas in a series of free exchanges between mother and baby. A healthy 4-month-old infant, for example, often has no difficulty showing focused attentiveness, particularly to the mothers' face and voice; using this focused attentiveness to be relaxed or calm; contributing to dependency by holding and finding comfortable positions—the infant holds the mother's neck and even begins directing the mother toward the type of rhythmic movements or sensory experiences that are most comforting; evidencing pleasure and joy by smiling in synchrony with the mother's smile or vocalizations; showing assertiveness and curiosity by somewhat chaotically but purposefully moving both arms to grasp an object; expressing anger, frustration, or protest with a distinct cry, angry look, and a flailing of arms and legs when a desired object is taken away; evidencing negativism and even belligerency by refusing to open his or her mouth or by spitting up whatever is disliked. These affective-thematic dimensions, which are differentiated during the first and second year, have been partitioned by investigators into subcategories and subtle gradations. Interestingly, adaptive toddlers by 14 to 18 months of age appear to have all the "moves;" that is, they have subtle affective expressions, including bewilderment, surprise, anticipation, and even a little smirk as they deliberately behave provocatively or negatively. The disturbed toddler's emotions, in comparison, are somewhat global and dampened.

The type of experience a child evidences is, in a sense, the drama the child is experiencing, whereas the organizational level may be viewed metaphorically as the stage on which this drama is being played. To carry this metaphor a step further, it is possible to imagine some stages that are large and stable and therefore able to support a complex and intense drama. In comparison, other stages may be narrow or small and thus able to contain only a very restricted drama. Still other stages may have cracks in them because of earlier faulty experience carried over into next phases, which then can crumble easily under the pressure of an intense, rich, and varied drama.

At each phase of development, there are certain characteristics that define the experiential organizational capacity; that is, the stability and contour of the stage. At the same time, there are certain age-appropriate dramas or themes characterized by their own complexity, richness, depth, and content. This type of developmental approach then provides a set of expectations and clinical-indicator behaviors or capacities for each age or developmental stage. It focuses on adaptive capacities expected, as well as on limitations and conflicts.

With this brief background, it is possible to identify areas of children's functioning, where either how they organize experience, or the particular content of their experience, requires further understanding. The volume, *The Feeling Child,* makes a major contribution to both these domains. The excellent articles in this volume on aspects of children's emotional development and coping and the factors which influence them, all have a common thread, to understand those experiences of the growing child (in the context of his or her family and culture) that are special because they have emotional meaning.

"The Role of Emotions in Development," by Michael Lewis, presents compelling reasons for balancing the current over-focus on cognition. Maria Piers and Nancy Curry present a broad overview on the development of emotional life, followed by a detailed review of the affective development literature by Janet Strayer. Especially valuable is Gil Foley's insights into the special challenges handicapped infants and their families face in establishing mutually pleasurable, meaningful emotional interaction patterns. How parents can turn the passive experience of T.V. watching into an active learning experience is analyzed by Jerome L. Singer and Dorothy Singer.

Putting our new understanding of infants and children into therapeutic contexts is instructively discussed by Nancy Curry (in terms of a model of play and language), Victoria Jean Dimidjian (in terms of a social family model of coping), and by Hugo Crago (in terms of an extremely interesting approach to how imagination and story telling both reveal and help to solve emotional conflicts).

As can be seen, this is an exciting volume which makes an important contribution to our perspectives on infants and children. Emotional development is not only important; it must be valued as cognitive achievements are. There is now an enormous amount of research and a variety of useful developmental models of emotional life, and these new models and insights of the organization and content of children's inner worlds can be applied in a range of normative, educational, and therapeutic settings.

REFERENCES

Greenspan, S. I. (1979). Intelligence and adaptation: An integration of psychoanalytic and Piagetian developmental psychology. *Psychological Issues, Vol. 12* (3/4), Monograph 47/48. New York: International Universities Press.

Greenspan, S. I. & Greenspan, N. T. (1985). *First Feelings: Milestones in the Emotional Development of the Infant and Young Child.* New York: Viking Penguin, Inc.

Greenspan, S. I. & Lourie, R. S. (1981). Developmental Structuralist Approach to the Classification of Adaptive and Pathologic Personality Organizations: Infancy and Early Childhood. *American Journal of Psychiatry, 138*(6), pp. 725–735.

THEORETICAL PERSPECTIVES

The Role of Emotion in Development

Michael Lewis, PhD

ABSTRACT. The study of emotional behavior has been slow, in part, based on Western societies view that emotional development is less important than cognitive development. In this paper we review the issue of the importance of emotional development for the young child. It is agreed that emotional well being may be as important as cognitive growth in determining life outcomes. Data from a variety of sources are reviewed and indicate cognitive skills, physical health and emotional well being *all* are necessary and constitute important goals for our children.

INTRODUCTION

The reciprocal roles of cognition in emotion and emotion in cognition are topics of recent interest (Lazarus, 1982; Lewis, Sullivan, & Michalson, 1984; Zajonc, 1980). It is not our aim here to address this connection, rather we wish instead to argue for the need to address the imbalance between the concern for cognition at the expense of emotion.

Michael Lewis, is Professor of Pediatrics, Psychiatry and Psychology; Chief of the Division of Child Development, Rutgers Medical School, Medical Education Building CN19, New Brunswick, NJ 08903. This paper was supported in part by a grant from the W. T. Grant Foundation.

We restrict our discussion to emotional development recognizing that the distinction between emotional, cognitive or social can be quite arbitrary. Indeed, any specific behavior might be considered to reflect any one of these dimensions. For example, research on facial emotional expressions may reflect both emotional and cognitive processes. Piaget relied on emotional behaviors such as interest, surprise and joy to reflect on the cognitive structures of children (Haviland, 1976). Surprise or astonishment is another emotional variable often used to assess cognitive ability. For instance, Charlesworth (1969) used surprise at the disappearance of an object to judge the infant's understanding of object permanence. In a similar fashion, the emotions of curiosity and anger can be used to measure understanding or knowledge, and examples are to be found throughout Piaget's descriptions of his experiments with his children (Piaget, 1954). It should be clear from these brief illustrations that the inferences drawn about children's intellectual ability are closely tied to the observations of classes of their behavior that include motor and emotional aspects. Without either set of behaviors, it would be more difficult to deduce which mental structures are available to a young child, especially during the prelinguistic stage of development.

EMOTIONAL DEVELOPMENT IN LITERATURE

Since the 1930s, the study of emotion and emotional development has been relatively stagnant, until quite recently, when there has been a renewal of interest and research in this area. In examining some of the more prominent child psychology textbooks (Carmichael, 1946, 1954; Jersild, 1933; Mussen, 1970; Mussen, Conger & Kagan, 1979; Osofsky, 1979), one finds that the page allotment to emotional topics is and always has been rather sparse.

We have undertaken topical analysis of the differences in page allocations in various textbooks. Recognizing the somewhat arbitrary nature of the classification system, one can still see that there have been few changes over the last 50 years in the percentage of pages devoted to emotional topics. For instance, in the 1930s, Murchison (1933) and Jersild (1933) devoted between 4% and 15% of their pages to emotional topics while in the 1970s Osofsky (1979), Mussen (1970), and Mussen et al. (1979) devoted 10%, 8%, and 7%, respectively. Compared with the coverage of perceptual-cognitive topics, the space devoted to emotional topics is meager. Furthermore, this lack of balance between emotional and perceptual-cognitive discussions is apparent across time and applies to each of the volumes surveyed. Although the selection of textbooks is neither exhaustive nor random, this survey underscores the relatively minor role given to emotional topics in the past.

Even within the discussions of emotion, the scope of coverage is limited in terms of the kinds of emotions discussed. When one examines the same sample of textbooks, it becomes obvious that more emphasis is given to negative emotions than to positive emotions. There is more written on sorrow, gloom, and sadness than on laughter and humor and more on jealousy than on sympathy. Without question, the most lengthy discussions have concentrated on fear, anger, and aggression. In every textbook surveyed, one or more of these feelings were allotted the largest number of pages.

Although we have quantified our survey of child psychology textbooks, one would need only to glance at the shelves in any psychology library to discover that of the books written about emotions, the vast majority are on aggression and hostility. Other topics represented, in descending order of frequency, include anxiety, shyness, fear, bereavement and grief, jealousy, laughter and humor, loneliness, and love. Even the number of words in the English language referring to negative emotions is significantly greater than the number of words referring to positive emotions, even though among nonemotional concepts, positive terms outnumber negative ones (Averill, 1980).

More recently, however, issues related to positive emotions have occupied an increasing number of pages in child psychology textbooks. For example, in the volumes edited by Osofsky (1979) and Mussen (1970), attachment topics are given either the most or the second most number of pages compared with other feeling states. And while jealousy receives more attention than sympathy, the recent work on empathy and role taking may alter this balance (Hoffman, 1978; Masangkay, McCluskey, McIntyre, Sims-Knight, Vaughn, & Flavell, 1974).

These data do not tell the entire story, however. Significant contributions to emotion theory have been made in the past two decades by investigators such as Tomkins (1962, 1963), Ekman (Ekman, Friesen, & Ellsworth, 1972); (Lewis & Brooks-Gunn, 1979; Lewis & Michalson, 1982a, b, c,; Lewis & Michalson, 1983); Izard (1971, 1977); Plutchik (1970, 1980a, b); Arnold (1960); Sroufe (1979b); Emde (Emde, Gaensbauer, & Harmon, 1976) and Campos (Campos & Stenberg, 1981; Goldsmith & Campos, 1982). Nevertheless, issues related to cognitive theory and cognitive development continue to permeate the zeitgeist and capture the interests of most scientists.

EMOTIONS AND RELATED ISSUES

This concern with cognition as the most important aspect of development also manifests itself in measures of individual differences in development. Almost all of the current measures of children's developmental status are based on cognitive variables (Lewis, 1976, 1984). These measures are used not only to assess children but also to plan treatment programs and to evaluate intervention outcomes. Thus, not only do scientists tend to study cognition at the expense of other aspects of human behavior, but public policy and decision-making actions are determined by this activity as well. Although it has been shown repeatedly that all cultural activities, including scientific pursuits, are influenced by and influence the zeitgeist (Kuhn, 1970), it is still somewhat surprising that individual differences in cognitive ability remain the most important determinant of social policy. It is particularly surprising when social policy pertains to infants and young children, since most existing measures of cognitive ability designed for children during the first years of life are generally not very reliable or valid (Lewis & Fox, in press). Given the force of a prevailing zeitgeist, however, it is small wonder that few useful measures of individual differences other than cognitive ones have been developed or used to assess children's development, to initiate intervention programs, or to evaluate outcomes.

Perceptions With Cognition

Why did such a role for cognition emerge and remain dominant? Zigler and Trickett (1978) suggested that the use of the IQ as a measure in the evaluation of childhood intervention programs became popular because standard IQ tests are well-developed instruments that are easily administered and that relate to other behaviors of theoretical and practical significance. A more detailed analysis of this problem is too far removed from our present concerns to be covered here, although the problem must be addressed eventually in as much as the development of a new instrument must compete in the public arena with existing cognitive instruments.

The success of our venture may be judged more by current cultural values than by its worth from a scientific point of view. Anderson and Messick (1974) were among the first to issue an appeal to broaden the definition of competence to include more than cognitive components. More recently, social competence rather than IQ has been cited by Zigler and Trickett (1978) as a more important source of individual differences and a more powerful influence on public policy: "Social competence, rather than IQ, should be employed as the major measure of the success of intervention programs such as Head Start" (p. 793). "Social competence must reflect the success of the human being in meeting societal expectancies. . . . These measures of social competence should reflect something about the self-actualization or personal development of the human being" (p. 795). Greenspan (1980), as well, suggested that the critical aspects of competence might be temperament, character, and social awareness, each of which involves factors similar or related to emotional processes. Finally, Scarr (1981) has proposed that the term intellectual competence be used in assessing children's school abilities. Her notion of intellectual competence includes the cognitive, motivational, and social aspects of what Zigler (1979) called "social competence." The motivational and adjustment aspects of such an assessment clearly overlap with the affective domain.

From a scientific point of view, there is relatively little reason to base public policy decisions, intervention strategies, and assessment procedures on cognitive rather than social or emotional bases. Thus, whether we agree on the particular measure of competence, such as IQ cognitive level, educational achievement, motivational and emotional variables, or even physical health, the need to broaden our measurement interests to include various aspects of children's abilities is vital.

While we cannot pretend to know the cause of the preoccupation with cognition, it appears that deep-seated in our child-rearing system is a belief that intellectual development in children is highly related to and may even ensure their success as adults. When parents are questioned about what they want for their children, four major goals usually emerge. Parents, regardless of the children's age, typically want their children to be happy, healthy, successful, and intelligent. Notice that the goals include physical health, career success, and happiness, as well as wisdom. These categories are not unlike those mentioned by Zigler (1979) under the rubric of social competence.

Underlying these four goals is the general premise that being smart (having highly developed intellectual skills) will ultimately lead to the other goals. In other words, most of us subscribe to the argument that cognitive abilities (usually in the form of academic achievement or IQ) are directly related to the acquisition of wealth, happiness, and physical health, as well as to the absence of psychopathology.

Although the data do not support this model (McClelland, 1973), it has become and remains a predominant theme in social policy. For example, one of the early assumptions of the Head Start program was that if we make children smarter, we will make them happier and more successful and will at the same time eliminate problems of social disorganization such as juvenile delinquency, truancy, alcoholism, and drug abuse (Hellmuth, 1968). Zigler himself has now challenged this premise: "Stated most simply, we believe that one can obtain a very high IQ score and still not behave admirably in the real world that exists beyond the confines of the psychologist's testing room" (Zigler & Trickett, 1978, p. 791).

Emotional Development and Later Occupation

Empirical evidence suggests that cognitive variables, such as grades in school and academic ability, are not good predictors of future success (McClelland, 1973). This finding seems to be true for jobs ranging from factory worker, bank teller, or air traffic controller (Berg, 1970) to scientific researcher (Taylor, Smith & Ghiselin, 1963). Jencks (1972) noted that while a person's occupation may be related to the amount of education received (insofar as educational background enables one to enter the occupation initially), when the effects of education are statistically controlled, the relationship between childhood IQ and later occupation all but disappears. Aptitude test scores seem to be no better at predicting later success than are school grades or IQ (McClelland, 1973).

In studies showing that scores on general intelligence tests correlate with proficiency across jobs (Ghiselli, 1966), the effects of social-class background or of personal credentials are seldom taken into account. It is fairly well established that social-class background is related to getting higher scores on ability tests (Nuttal & Fozard, 1970), as well as to having the right personal credentials for success. Consequently, the relationship between aptitude or intelligence and job success is likely to be illusory, a product of their joint association with social class.

Intelligence measures, then, do not seem to predict successful job performance very well. They also bear little relationship to later earnings (Duncan, Featherman, & Duncan, 1972; Jencks, 1972). Likewise, within a given occupation, academic credentials do not have much effect on income, although such credentials, as we pointed out earlier, may be related to the occupation entered. Family background seems to be more related to income levels than either IQ scores or academic variables (Jencks, 1972).

Emotional Development and Life Adjustment

If cognitive and intellectual measures do not predict a person's later career success or wealth with much accuracy, what about happiness and health? If we make children smarter, will they be healthier and happier, if not wealthier and wiser? Does intellectual ability promote better adjustment to life as is often claimed? In independent studies, Jensen (1972) and Kohlberg, LaCrosse, and Ricks (1970) examined longitudinal data from a sample of gifted individuals and concluded that the gifted experience more occupational, marital, and social success than nongifted individuals and have lower incidences of alcoholism and homosexuality. However, the data were based on Terman and Oden's (1947) study, in which no attempt was made to equate for the opportunity to achieve success. The gifted subjects came from socio-economic backgrounds superior to those of the nongifted subjects. Again, a failure to take into account social class and all that it entails such as educational advantages, job contacts, and occupational credentials may result in spuriously high correlations between intelligence and success. Finally, satisfaction with one's job does not appear to be related to educational attainment (Jencks, 1972), nor is there evidence that intelligence is related to less neuroticism (McClelland, 1973).

Given the disappointing showing of cognitive measures in explaining career success, job earnings, or satisfaction with life, one might want to consider altering the past assumptions. Perhaps life's outcomes are more influenced by "happiness" than by cognitive skills. If Zigler is correct that self-actualization or personal development may be a more important source of individual differences, then emotional and motivational variables may be the causal factors in a successful and intellectually rewarding life. Jencks (1972) found that noncognitive attributes seem to play a larger role than cognitive skills in determining career success or failure. In particular, whether the subject stayed in school, it was found to predict later income as well as test scores, and to predict occupation status better than test scores did.

Emotional Development and Intellectual Development

Although there are few data on the subject, there is some reason to believe that emotional variables also play an important role in children's early intellectual development. For example, "personality traits" may be more predictive of later cognitive growth than earlier measures of cognitive difference. In a study of the predictive value of both earlier IQ scores and the degree of pleasure or happiness the child showed in taking the test, Birns and Golden (1972) found that the happiness rating was far more predictive of later IQ scores than was the earlier IQ measure. There is also evidence that early differences in emotional response predict later adaptation and competence. In particular, positive affect during play at 18 months has been shown to predict competence in a peer group at 3-1/2 years of age (Waters, Wippman & Sroufe, 1979). Positive affect and enthusiasm at 24 months seem to be related to measures of adaptation at 5 years (Arend, Gove, & Sroufe, 1979). Finally, Scarr (1981) has reported that being cooperative, attentive, less active, socially responsive, and well adjusted at 2 years of age is as predictive of higher IQ scores at 4 years as having a higher IQ score at 2 is predictive of being well-motivated to learn at 4.

The argument is also apparent in the work on attachment and exploration as it relates to the role of emotions in effecting intellectual development. Attachment can be viewed as an emotional or affectional tie between two people, in most cases between child and parent. It can also be viewed in its functional role, namely, that of providing a secure base from which children can explore their environment (Ainsworth & Bell, 1970). Given children's need (indeed, the need of all organisms) for exploration and novelty as well as the concurrent need for predictability and familiarity, attachment is conceptualized as the mechanism for providing the affective capacity for this duality of experience (Sroufe, 1979a). Through the establishment of reciprocal and responsive interactions and the emergence of a sense of self, children are able to establish relationships that, among other things, provide them with a secure base from which to explore their environment (Lewis & Brooks-Gunn, 1979). The underlying feeling state associated with attachment relationships is one of love and security. From this feeling state, infants are able to develop a variety of other competencies, including the abilities to explore, to relate to peers, and to maintain ego resiliency (Arend et al., 1979). Ainsworth and her colleagues (Ainsworth, Blehar, Waters, & Wall, 1978); Lewis et al. 1984 have also argued convincingly for the interface between this feeling state and children's commerce with the environment, a commerce that includes emotional as well as cognitive components.

Whereas attachment and the relationship of attachment to cognition have received some attention in the research literature, the feeling states of competence and efficacy and their relationship to performance have received more attention. White (1975, 1978; White & Watts, 1973), Lewis (Lewis & Goldberg, 1969b; Lewis & Coates 1980; Coates & Lewis,

1984), and Seligman (1975) have argued that feelings of competence and power and the reciprocal feeling of learned helplessness are important determinants of other skills and capacities often considered cognitive in nature. For example, infants who receive more contingent responses to their actions (presumably, infants who feel more competent) have more efficient exploration skills (Lewis & Goldberg, 1969b). These infants show faster habituation to redundant information than do infants who feel less competent.

Even more striking are the results from a recent study in our laboratory in which children 10–24 weeks of age were placed in two groups (Lewis, Sullivan, & Brooks-Gunn, 1985). In one group, infants' arm-pulling behavior resulted in the appearance of a picture. The second group served as a yoked control that received the same amount of stimulation but had no control over the appearance of a picture. It was hypothesized that control of the environment, that is, feelings of efficacy, would produce alterations in the infants' emotional state. Specifically, we predicted that competent infants would be more likely to show positive affect (smiling) and to stay awake and alert longer than powerless infants. Indeed, the results suggested that the infants who were able to control their environment were likely to stay awake longer and were less likely to cry than the infants who were equally stimulated but who were not in control of the stimulus.

A further example of the role of emotions in promoting success comes from research on the effects of anxiety on intellectual performance and educational achievement. The relationship between this feeling state and performance is not linear. Large and small amounts of anxiety may seriously affect cognitive as well as motor performance, whereas moderate amounts of anxiety may be facilitating (Sarason, 1980).

Emotional Development and Health

There is an accumulating body of evidence showing that emotions can affect physical health as well (Cherry, 1980). For example, there appears to be a direct link between a person's feelings and the body's immunological system. Negative emotions especially, such as anger and anxiety, may lower a crucial biological threshold and increase the risk of infection. Furthermore, manipulation of emotional states by means of biofeedback or medication may diminish physical pain and enhance one's general sense of well-being, as well as prevent sickness (Benson, 1975).

Other medical research suggests that personality traits may contribute to the development of heart disease and cancer. Much publicity has been devoted to the link between heart disease and the "Type A" personality, characterized by behaviors such as irritation, impatience, frustration, and anger (Friedman & Rosenman, 1974; Glass, 1977). The link between personality and cancer is somewhat more tenuous. There is some evidence that cancer patients who appear to be "model adults" (conscientious and dutiful) have experienced a disturbed childhood, filled with loneliness and hurt. Their stoicism as adults, in fact, hides a basic despair, and within a short time after a spouse dies or a job is lost, the first symptoms of cancer may appear (LeShan, 1977). Findings from a study of cancer in identical twins suggests that the twin who died of leukemia was the one who had experienced an emotional upheaval. Additional evidence of a link between emotions and cancer comes from a longitudinal study of more than a thousand graduates of Johns Hopkins University in which the subjects who developed major cancers were reported to be low-key, nonaggressive people, not close to their parents.

Not only is it possible that negative emotions, such as grief or anger, may contribute to heart disease and cancer, but positive emotions may actually prevent or cure physical illness (LeShan, 1980). In a personal account about the effects of a progressive and painful illness of the connective tissues, Cousins (1979) reported that 10 minutes of laughter (in response to Marx Brothers' movies) relieved his pain. Given about 1 in 500 chances of recovery, 16 years later Cousins reported that through laughter and humor, he was without pain and able to engage in sports.

A longitudinal study of 100 Harvard students showed that of these students judged to have the best mental health during college, only 2 had become seriously ill or died by the age of 53. Nearly half of those considered less well adjusted had fallen ill or died by their early 50's (Vaillant, 1977). Similarly, a longitudinal study of medical school graduates found evidence that only a quarter of the subjects judged to be either calm and stable or lively and flexible had endured a heart attack or cancer, compared to over three-quarters of a group of moody, irritable persons (Cherry, 1980). It seems, then, that both negative and positive emotions play a role in physical health. A word of caution is in order, however. It must be recognized that the role of emotions in physical health is likely to be modified by temperamental and environmental factors.

I have argued, elsewhere (Lewis & Michalson 1983), that in order to understand development, scientists must move away from the preoccupation with cognitive variables and redirect their attention to emotional development. We challenge the assumption that by increasing the cognitive abilities of children, we are ensuring their later success and happiness in life. Instead, we have presented studies showing that cognitive variables such as grades in school, IQ, and achievement test results do not predict occupational status, earnings, job satisfaction, or life adjustments. Indeed, there is some evidence that "emotional" variables, such as feelings of security, of pleasure in doing a task, or of competence, may have a more powerful influence on children's development. While the effort to determine which is more important, cognition or emotion, may be futile, we must, nevertheless, broaden our perspective of development, placing more evidence on emotional behavior and development than in the past.

ASSESSING EMOTIONAL DEVELOPMENT

In order to study children's emotions, it is necessary that we have a working theory of development as well as an assessment instrument for measuring emotional development. Even though in the past few years researchers have returned to the study of emotion, this area of inquiry is still plagued by the difficulties of measuring emotions in infants and young children. Despite the relatively large number of standardized instruments available for assessing cognitive development, emotional measures are scarce. The existing scales are usually restricted to measures of a single emotion or are appropriate for use only with older children. Tests for infants are generally used to gather descriptive data regarding the age of appearance of particular skills or behaviors. The few instruments that do include emotional variables tend to rely on subjective rating techniques to assess either general emotional tone (i.e., positive or negative affect) or general social adjustment. In addition, rather narrow measures of single emotional states have been taken in laboratory situations. While such studies may provide interesting data on children's emotions, the usefulness of laboratory experiments in understanding development in real-life settings has been repeatedly questioned (Riegel & Meacham, 1976). Unfortunately, much of contemporary developmental psychology can be described as "the science of the strange behavior of children in strange situations with strange adults for the briefest possible period of time" (Bronfenbrenner, 1977, p. 513).

In order to meet this challenge, Lewis & Michalson (1983) have constructed and utilized a Scale of Socio-emotional Development (SSD) which has proven useful for the (1) study of individual differences in emotional profiles, (2) age changes in emotional development, and (3) setting differences in emotional training. This last aspect refers to developing different emotional profiles as a part of day care curriculum. We have found that our scales are also helpful in changing and evaluating intervention programs. Our hope is that the development of a measurement instrument will allow us to consider emotions as an important aspect in the developing child and to measure individual differences in this domain. Given a measurement procedure, we hope to encourage others to consider empirically the emotional developmental process and its perturbations. Only then and in combination with cognitive and social measures can we say we have some understanding of the developmental process.

REFERENCES

Ainsworth, M. D. S., & Bell, S. M. (1970). Attachment, exploration, and separation illustrated by the behavior of one-year-olds in a strange situation. *Child Development, 41,* 49–67.

Ainsworth, M. D. S., Blehar, M., Waters, E., & Wall, S. (1978). *Patterns of attachment: A Psychological study of the strange situation.* Hillsdale, NJ: Erlbaum.

Anderson, J. & Messick, S. (1974). Social competency in young children. *Developmental Psychology, 10,* 282–293.

Arend, R., Gove, F. L., & Sroufe, L. A. (1979). Continuity of individual adaptation from infancy to kindergarten: A predictive study of ego resiliency and cuiriosity in preschoolers. *Child Development, 50,* 950–959.

Arnold, M. B. (1960). *Emotion and personality* (2 Vols.). New York: Columbia University Press.

Averill, J. R. (1980). On the paucity of positive emotions. In K. R. Blankstein, P. Pliner, & J. Polivy (Eds.), *Assessment and modification of emotional behavior.* New York: Plenum.

Benson, H. (1975). *The relaxation response.* New York: Morrow.

Berg, I. (1970). *Education and jobs: The great training robbery.* New York: Praeger.

Birns, B., & Golden, M. (1972). Prediction of intellectual performance at 3 years from infant tests and personality measures. *Merrill-Palmer Quarterly, 18,* 53–58.

Bronfenbrenner, V. (1977). Toward an experimental ecology of human development. *American Psychologist, 32,* 513–531.

Carmichael, L. (Ed.). (1946). *Manual of child psychology.* New York: Wiley.

Carmichael, L. (Ed.). (1954). *Manual of child psychology* (2nd Ed.). New York: Wiley.

Campos, J., & Stenberg, C. (1981). Perception, appraisal, and emotion: The onset of social referencing. In M. E. Lamb & L. R. Sherrod (Eds.), *Infant Social Cognition: Empirical and Theoretical considerations.* Hillsdale, NJ: Erlbaum.

Charlesworth, W. R. (1969). The role of surprise in cognitive development. In D. Elkind & J. H. Flavell (Eds.), *Studies in cognitive development: Essays in honor of Jean Piaget.* London: Oxford University Press.

Cherry, L. (1980, November 23). How the mind affects our health. *The New York Times Magazine,* p. 24.

Coates, D., & Lewis, M. (1984). Early mother-infant interaction and infant cognitive status as predictors of school performance and cognitive behavior in six year olds. *Child Development,* 1219–1230.

Cousins, N. (1979). *Anatomy of an illness as perceived by the patient: Reflections in healing and regeneration.* New York: Norton.

Duncan, O. D., Featherman, D. L., & Duncan, B. (1972). *Socioeconomic background and achievement.* New York: Seminar Press.

Ekman, P., Friesen, W. V., & Ellsworth, P. (1972). *Emotion in the human face: Guidelines for research and an integration of findings.* New York: Pergamon.

Emde, R. N., Gaensbauer, T., & Harmon, R. (1976). Emotional expression in infancy: A biobehavioral study. *Psychological Issues, 10,* (1, Whole No. 37).

Friedman, M., & Rosenman, R. H. (1974). *Type A behavior and your heart.* New York: Knopf.

Ghiselli, E. E. (1966). *The validity of occupational aptitude tests.* New York: Wiley.

Glass, D. C. (1977). *Behavior patterns, stress, and coronary disease.* New York: Erlbaum.

Goldsmith, H., & Campos, J. J. (1982). Toward a theory of infant temperament. In R. Emde & R. Harmon (Eds.), *Attachment and affiliative systems.* New York: Plenum Press.

Greenspan, S. (1980). Is social competence synonymous with school performance? *American Psychologist, 35,* 938–939.

Haviland, J. (1976). Looking smart: The relationship between affect and intelligence in infancy. In M. Lewis (Ed.), *Origins of Intelligence: Infancy and early childhood* (pp. 423–449). New York: Plenum Press.

Hellmuth, J. (Ed.). (1968). *Disadvantaged child: Head Start and early intervention.* New York: Brunner/Mazel.

Hoffman, M. L. (1978). Empathy, its development and prosocial implications. In H. E. Howe, Jr. & C. B. Keasey (Eds.), *Nebraska symposium on motivation* (vol. 25). Lincoln: University of Nebraska Press.

Izard, C. E. (1971). *The face of emotion.* New York: Appleton.

Izard, C. E. (1971). *Human emotions.* New York: Plenum.

Jencks, C. (1972). *Inequality: A reassessment of the effect of family and schooling* .. *America.* New York: Basic Books.

Jensen, A. R. (1972). The heritability of intelligence. *Saturday Evening Post,* 244, (2), 9.

Jersild, A. T. (1933). *Child psychology.* New York: Prentice-Hall.

Kohlberg, L., LaCrosse, J., & Ricks, D. (1970). The predictability of adult mental health from childhood behavior. In B. Wolman (Ed.), *Handbook of child psychopathology.* New York: McGraw-Hill.

Kuhn, T. S. (1970). *The structure of scientific revolution* (2nd ed.). Chicago: University of Chicago Press.

Lazarus, R. S. (1982). Thoughts on the relations between emotion and cognition. *American Psychologist, 37,* 1019–1024.

LeShan, L. (1977). *You can fight for your life: Emotional factors in the causation of cancer.* New York: Evans.

LeShan, L. (1980). *You can fight for your life: Emotional factors in the treatment of cancer.* New York: Evans.

Lewis, M. (1976). *Origins of intelligence: Infancy and early childhood.* New York: Plenum Press.

Lewis, M., & Brooks-Gunn, J. (1979). *Social cognition and the acquisition of self.* New York: Plenum Press.

Lewis, M., & Coates, D. L. (1980). Monther-infant interaction and cognitive development in 12-week-old infants. *Infant Behavior and Development, 3,* 95–105.

Lewis, M., Feiring, C., McGuffog, C., & Jaskir, J. (1984). Predicting psychopathology in six year olds from early social relations. *Child Development, 55,* 123–136.

Lewis, M., & Fox, N. (in press). Infant assessment: Challenges for the future. In M. Lewis (Ed.), *Prenatal and perinatal factors relevant to learning disabilities.* University of Illinois Press.

Lewis, M., & Goldberg, S. (1969b). Perceptual-cognitive development in infancy: A generalized expectancy model as a function of the mother-infant interaction. *Merrill-Palmer Quarterly, 16,* 81–100.

Lewis, M., & Michalson, L. (1982a). *From emotional state to emotional expression.* Paper presented at the symposium on Human Development from the Perspective of Person and Environment Interactions, University of Stockholm, Stockholm, Sweden, June.

Lewis, M., & Michalson, L. (1982b). The measurement of emotional state. In C. E. Izard (Ed.), *Measuring emotions in infants and children.* New York: Cambridge University Press.

Lewis, M., & Michalson, L. (1982c). The socialization of emotions. In T. Field & A. Fogel (Eds.), *Emotion and early interaction.* Hillsdale, New Jersey: Erlbaum.

Lewis, M., Michalson, L. (1983). *Children's emotions and moods: Developmental theory and measurement.* New York: Plenum Press.

Lewis, M., Sullivan, M., & Brooks-Gunn, J. (1985). Emotional behavior during the learning of a contingency in early infancy. *British Journal of Developmental Psychology, 3,* 307–316.

Masangkay, Z. S., McCluskey, K. A., McIntyre, C. W., Sims-Knight, J., Vaugn, B. E., & Flavell, J. H. (1974). The early development of inferences about the visual percepts of others. *Child Development, 45,* 357–366.

McClelland, D. C. (1973). Testing for competence rather than for "intelligence." *American Psychologist, 23,* 114.

Murchison, C. (Ed.). (1933). *A handbook of child psychology* (2nd ed., rev.) Worcester, Mass: Clark University Press.

Mussen, P. H. (Ed.). (1970). *Carmichael's manual of child psychology* (3rd ed., 2 vols). New York: Wiley.

Mussen, P. H., Conger, J. J., & Kagan, J. (1979). *Child development and personality* (5th ed.). New York: Harper & Row.

Nuttal, R. L., & Fozard, T. A. (1970). Age, Socioeconomic status and human abilities. *Aging and Human Development, 1,* 16–169.

Osofsky, J. D. (1979). *Handbook of infant development.* New York: Wiley.

Piaget, J. (1954). *Construction of reality in the child.* New York: Basic Books.

Plutchik, R. (1970). Emotions, evolution and adaptive processes. In M. Arnold (Ed.), *Feelings and emotions.* New York: Academic Press.

Plutchik, R. (1980a). *Emotion: A psychoevolutionary synthesis.* New York: Harper & Row.

Plutchik, R. (1980b). A general psychoevolutionary theory of emotion. In R. Plutchik & H. Kellerman (Eds.), *Emotion: Theory research, and experience.* New York: Academic Press.

Riegel, K., & Meacham, J. (Eds.). (1976). *The developing individual in a changing world,* Vol. 2: *Social and environmental issues.* The Hague: Mouton.

Sarason, I. G. (1980). *Test anxiety: Theory, research, and applications.* Hillsdale, New Jersey: Erlbaum.

Scarr, S. (1981). Testing for children: Assessment and the many determinants of intellectual competence. *American Psychologist, 36,* 1159–1166.

Seligman, M. E. P. (1975). *Helplessness: On depression, development, and death.* San Francisco: Freeman.

Sroufe, L. A. (1979a). The coherence of individual development: Early care, attachment and subsequent development issues. *American Psychologist, 34,* 834–841.

Sroufe, L. A. (1979b). Socioemotional development. In J. D. Osofsky (Ed.), *Handbook of infant development.* New York: Wiley.

Taylor, C., Smith, W. R., Ghiselin, B. (1963). The creative and other contributions of one sample of research scientists. In C. W. Taylor & F. Barron (Eds.), *Scientific Creativity: Its recognition and development.* New York: Wiley.

Terman, L. M., & Oden, M. H. (1947). *The gifted child grows up.* Stanford, California: Stanford University Press.

Tomkins, S. S. (1962). *Affect, imagery, consciousness: Vol. 1: The positive affects.* New York: Springer.

Tomkins, S. S. (1963). *Affect, imagery, consciousness: Vol. 2: The negative affect.* New York: Springer.

Vaillant, G. (1977). *Adaptation to life.* Boston: Little, Brown.

Waters, E., Wippman, J., & Sroufe, L. A. (1979). Attachment, positive affect, and competence in the peer group: Two studies in construct validation. *Child Development, 50,* 821–829.

White, B. L. (1975). Critical influences in the origins of competence. *Merrill-Palmer Quarterly, 21,* 243–266.

White, B. L. (1978). *Experience and Environment-Major influences on the development of young children* (Vol. 2). Englewood Cliffs, N.J.: Prentice-Hall.

White, B. L. & Watts, J. C. (1973). *Experience & environment: Major influence on the development of the young child* (vol 1). Englewood Cliffs, New Jersey: Prentice-Hall.

Zajonc, R. B. (1980). Feeling and thinking: Preferences need no inferences. *American Psychologist, 35,* 151–175.

Zigler, E. (1979). Project Head Start: Success or failure? In E. Zigler & J. Valentine (Eds.), *Project Head Start.* New York: Free Press.

Zigler, E., & Trickett, P. K. (1978). IQ, social competence, and evaluation of early childhood intervention programs. *American Psychologist, 33,* 789–798.

A Developmental Perspective on Children's Affects

Maria W. Piers, PhD, DHL
Nancy E. Curry, PhD

ABSTRACT. While it is a popular belief that affect is experienced only once organized thought begins, observation tells us differently. Newborn babies cry when they are uncomfortable, and their early smiles, after the first five weeks, are not merely reflexive, but an indication that infants feel good about something or somebody. After the first five months emotional responses become increasingly independent from physical pain or pleasure, and increasingly differentiated. Parents begin to play a lesser role in the lives and emotions of older preschoolers and school-age children. These children identify with their peers, whom they admire or resent strongly and from whom they feel compelled to learn. At all times, however, regardless of what they are learning and from whom, children are propelled by their affect. Therefore, any adult who deals with children must be aware of their emotions and use them to facilitate the child's acquisition of skills and knowledge.

INTRODUCTION

Jonah's parents spent the first years of their married life in a small college town in the midwest. It was there that Jonah was born and where he spent the first nine months of his life.

It was a peaceful existence. Since both parents were employed on the campus, there was a third adult who took care of Jonah. Peter, a graduate student in psychology, was the regular babysitter. He sat with the little boy

---

Maria W. Piers is Distinguished Service Professor Erikson Institute, Chicago, Illinois 60610. Nancy E. Curry is Professor and Program Director, Child Development and Child Care, School of Health Related Professions, University of Pittsburgh 15260.

for a number of hours every day, and he and Jonah became very fond of each other. Then, when Jonah was nine months old, the family moved to a different campus following a better job opportunity and Jonah's friendship with Peter was rudely interrupted. Not that Jonah seemed to mind. His mother had more time for him in the new location, and Jonah developed into a cheerful and active toddler.

One day, Jonah's parents received a letter from Peter in which he announced his impending visit to their new home. He missed Jonah and decided to visit his former charge. It was their first encounter after 21 months. Both Peter and Jonah smiled politely by way of a greeting, but then Jonah did something quite extraordinary. He got down on all fours and repeated all the little games he had played with Peter in the good old days, which he had since outgrown: games like finger games, and peek-a-boo. Peter, of course, complied, and the silent dialogue of reminiscing went on for a while.

But then Jonah put his hand on Peter's knee and said clearly and urgently "backpack," referring to his once favorite mode of transportation, for which at nine months he did not yet have that word. In time, then, Jonah had acquired and properly used the term for a most pleasurable experience of long ago. Thus Jonah demonstrated the fact that human beings feel strongly, and recall those feelings, from very early on. Strangely, this is hard for many nonprofessional persons to believe. "But how could Jonah remember that Peter had carried him around in a backpack when he was too young to think?" The answer is that a memory is often evoked (perhaps even invariably) by the affect experienced at the time.

This vignette illustrates what Kernberg (1978) refers to as "affective memory" (p. 339). Affective memory incorporated Jonah's feeling state with his self-image which clearly began to include internalized aspects of this important person in his life. In addition, the vignette illustrates the current psychoanalytic position concerning affects; that is, that they both demonstrate and serve as an organizational process in the developing child (Emde, 1980) and are nurtured and differentiated through meaningful relationships with other people (Kernberg, 1978).

The upsurge of interest in affective development is evidenced in recent books which report data from both psychologists (e.g., Lewis and Michalson, 1983) and psychoanalysts (e.g., Emde, Gaensbauer and Harmon, 1976). Greenspan and Greenspan (1985) have just written a sorely needed book for parents tracing the emotional milestones in children from birth through age four. Strayer's review article in this issue further attests to the renewed interest in this area. The current research seems to support the clinical findings that psychoanalysts and others working with children have noted over the years. This paper will deal with elaboration of affects in the young child from birth to school-age. The role of caregivers in aiding in the differentiation of affects and behavioral manifestations of certain affects will be considered from a psychoanalytic perspective as enhanced by some recent relevant empirical studies.

Infancy

Returning to the vignette about Jonah, it seems clear that it is positive affect that seems to make life worth living for a small infant. Conversely, it is the absence of such a positive affect that can be seen in all "failure to thrive" babies. This is clearly shown in Spitz's (1983) hospitalism study, in Provence and Lipton's study (1962) of institutionalized children and in the work of the Rochester group which has delineated the roots of helplessness in early infancy (Schmale, 1964). It is also shown in the recent work of Field, Woodson, Greenberg and Cohen (1982) with newly born infants as they imitate with a great sense of urgency the facial expression of the person who makes eye-contact with them. Tronick, Ricks and Cohn (1982) also report on the marked effect mothers' simulated depression had on their older babies, even when simulation was for a brief period of time.

Is "feeling good" then a physical state or an emotional one? For a small child there is no difference between the two. Hoffer (1950) speaks of the "body ego" which refers to the locus of feelings and experiences centering on the child's body. As Mahler and McDevitt (1980) state, "Maturational process and maternal care together bring about in the infant an increased sensory awareness of his body's periphery, along with a progressive sensory awareness of the outer world" (p. 398). Through predictable and loving caregiving, the baby becomes aware of what feelings come from inside himself or herself and what comes to him or her from the external world. This brings about self-awareness and an awareness of the important caregivers.

Nevertheless, throughout the first year, pleasure and displeasure are experienced physically. Physical discomfort is tantamount to emotional misery and pleasant affect is tantamount to physical well-being. It is only later in life, though it is hard to say exactly when, that we are capable of feeling happy even though we are suffering from a physical discomfort such as a fractured leg, or conversely that we are depressed even though the doctor has just told us there is nothing physically wrong with us.

As for Jonah and Peter, it is of course possible that their friendship was pure and cloudless, that they were just happy together, but it is not very likely. For in most relationships between adults and children an occasional bit of anger or disappointment must fall. In fact, frustrations are a necessary challenge in order to help children grow. The inevitable frustrations imposed result in many conflicts of interest between the generations. It is, however, true that in a child's memory one or the other impression prevails: either Mom appears all kind and good because the most recent memory is the distribution of ice cream cones, or else Mom is remembered as all mean because she sternly states, "No more ice cream cones today." It is hard for us to guess whether the "good" mother will leave the predominant impression, or the "bad" mother will. This all or nothing attitude toward the caregiver seems to exist throughout the first year of life, and continues into the next. Experts frequently refer to this phenomenon as the "splitting of the parent image." (Kernberg, 1978; Kohut, 1971).

In terms of affective development during the first year, Erikson (1950) in describing the normal crises that occur epigenetically throughout the life cycle, has spoken of the sense of *trust* versus that of *mistrust* developed in the first year; Benedek (1938) used the label of *confident expectation.* These global affective labels proved to be useful constructs in describing primary affective states which become part of one's personality development throughout life. Psychoanalysts and psychiatrists, however, are showing empirically that a wide variety of emotions (at least 10) can be discerned in infants through discriminative facial movements (Izard, 1979). Gaensbauer (1982), in utilizing Izard's coding system, found that "the capacity to express in at least rudimentary forms the emotions of joy, interest, fear, anger, and sadness, as well as the more undifferentiated emotion of distress, appears to be present by 4 months of age" (p. 51). By the end of the first year the child has a wide repertoire of emotional expressiveness, but still will have difficulty understanding and differentiating any ambiguous emotional intents of the primary caregiver.

Toddlerhood

One of the tasks of toddlerhood, then, is for the child to learn to view us as "just human," with some generous, warm attributes and competencies and some flaws as well. Mahler, Pine and Bergman (1975) feel that the child demonstrates this capacity upon the achievement of libidinal object constancy, that is, that one has a stable internalized image of the parents that enables one to acknowledge that they can be good and bad and still be the same persons. Until we achieve this realistic portrayal of our elders (and an achievement it is indeed), we remember our happy and unhappy feelings in accordance with the developmental stage during which they took place. Gradually, thereafter, our affect is not simply positive or negative, but becomes more and more differentiated. Bad feelings can be specifically sadness, anger, a mild unlust, passivity, disinterest, or an urge to attack or get even by way of a sit down strike or whatever. Equally differentiated are the causes that bring on a negative response. This is particularly true when a child feels a strong urge to smash a valued glass bowl, pull somebody's hair, or otherwise engage in destructive behavior. Obviously the nearest responsible adult will stop him.

Things are, however, more complicated when two opposing

tendencies arise from within a little boy or girl, rather than from a dilemma posed by someone in the environment. What if, for instance, Kenneth, age two, wants to assert himself by crayoning graffiti on the living room wall and at the same time wants to stay in his mother's good graces? Both just cannot be done. Mother will be angry at his artistic endeavor; knowing this reinforces his rage and makes him all the more "artistic." Undoubtedly, the rage of frustration is also reinforced by such circumstances as the incidental presence of a disliked babysitter, or the fact that the mudlike substance being prepared for a chocolate cake is deemed by Mother to be unsuitable for mudpies.

Erikson (1950) describes beautifully such quandaries of the willful toddler. The battles of will that must be fought at this stage leave either a lasting sense of autonomous self or an abiding sense of shame and doubt. Piers and Singer (1953) too note the occurrence of the roots of shame in this stage. More recently, Sander (1975) speaks of the adaptational issues which are confronted by toddlers as they move toward a solid sense of self. The last two issues are those of *recognition* and *continuity*. *Recognition* refers to the child's need to develop an inner awareness "of his own feelings, his fantasies, and his play objectives" (Sander 1979, p. 141). *Continuity* describes the child's sense of self-constancy of himself and the constancy of others regardless of the disruptions that occur because of the toddler's "intentionally destructive and directed acts of aggression" (p. 143).

Preschool

The differentiation of emotions that occurs during the first year, and the later consolidation of the sense of self, provide the young child forever after with a whole range of emotions. When a 3-year-old falls on the playground and injures his knee, the rage is not the only expression of strong emotion; it goes along with the expression of wonderful fun, or with tears. All the positive feelings can be expressed just as well. There is the giggle of surprise when children seem to outwit an adult, the laughter of mirth when daddy tickles them, or the quiet happy satisfaction because they successfully managed to put on their shoes.

Preschoolers can be exhilarated when they succeed in solving a cognitive task or a task requiring coordination. It seems in fact that throughout our lifetime most, if not all, cognitive and complex intellectual pursuits are accompanied by affect. It sounds like a cliche when we state that any problem which children are able to solve is bound to make them pleased or proud or indeed elated. White (1968) developed the concept of *affectance motivation,* which is characteristic of the child's seeking activities calculated to bring about effective changes in the environment. Problem solving increases the child's self-esteem. This self-esteem in turn is a driving force to seek solutions to new puzzles and to enjoy them as best one can.

Sometimes it is indeed difficult to tell if a game of counting buttons or jellybeans is accompanied primarily by the "aha" feeling and whether it is a happy or unhappy one, but the experience is always loaded with emotions. And such experiences can be primarily affective or cognitive, but most of the time they are some of both. When, for instance, a 4-year-old girl tells her mother "I'm going to marry my daddy and then we will tuck you in at 7:00 o'clock, and then daddy and I will go to the movies," it is immediately recognizable as a statement born out of a strong affect. It is not only affect. Little Susie is in love with her father and that affect poses any number of cognitive problems which she will have to solve (Fraiberg, 1959; Piers, 1966).

The imagination and conjecturing and the projecting into the future which are at every Susie's and Tommy's disposal, are limitless; and so are the varied feeling tones of joy and displeasure, as well as the capacity for guilt. It should, therefore, not surprise us if the Oedipal child under the impact of strong and incompatible feelings suffers from nightmares and other physiological manifestations of overwhelming affect. The fact that little Tommy loves and needs his father even while wishing that his daddy would die and never come back, leaving his privileged place at mother's side to his little son, seems a well-nigh insoluble problem. We, the grown-ups, know that, all things being equal, most Tommys and Susies do indeed reach the point where the positive affect of great love and the negative ones of intense hate reduce themselves to a mere competitive striving that does not call for tears, wakeful nights, or guilt feelings. At the same time, the fact that children become more skillful in every way makes for an increasing self-confidence (which is also an emotional experience) and a better relationship between father and son or mother and daughter.

Erikson (1950) refers to the polarities of this period as those of *initiative* vs. *guilt*. The Oedipal strivings of the preschooler involve much pleasure and pain but are modulated through the child's capacity for fantasy which is expressed in dramatic play, art, and other forms of world construction (Sutton-Smith, 1971). Gould's (1972) research supports our position that affect and cognition are intertwined and mutually effect one another. She reports that early experience and feelings surrounding nurturing and caregiving are reflected in the roles preschool children chose to play out, the style in which they approach fantasy play, and even their ability or inability to involve themselves in depthful, rewarding play episodes.

School-Age

As we know, most children as they move toward school-age do indeed resolve the Oedipal conflict and the ambivalent feelings that accompany it. Even so, there are often some residues, as shown in a certain irritability toward one parent, whereas the other parent is treated with much more patience or even empathy. It may be particularly evident when there is a switch during the early school years. The switch can be quite startling to parents. For instance, little Brian, who for the first five years of his life appeared to be particularly close to his mother, becomes unexpectedly an ally or even a defender of his father on occasions of marital disagreement which occurs in all families. It is as if Brian has reversed his allegiances. He is not mother's boy anymore; rather, he aims at being a man with men.

There are other shifts in the emotional climate of the school-age child. It is not just that the affect changes, but also that the persons to whom the child directs affects are different. Whereas the main love and longing as well as anger were previously directed toward the caring grownup, (i.e., parent or teacher), it is now increasingly important that one turn to one's peer group. Nevertheless adults continue to be important. The rage and anger that some children feel toward unloving, hurtful parents can get displaced onto well meaning teachers, who become discouraged and eventually avoid the very children who need their understanding if they are to be receptive to what the teacher has to offer.

Misunderstandings also can come about if we disregard fear and anger and the big role they play in learning. The fear of body damage that most early grade school children harbor was exacerbated by a first grade teacher who told her fellow teachers with glee of managing group discipline by threatening the children that she would "cut off your privileges." The children were indeed silent, but flooded with fear and unable to attend the task for which the teacher had subdued them.

During school-age years, we expect and usually witness the rapid increase in basic cognitive and motoric skills. At the same time, we must also recognize that a child's emotional responses must be taken seriously by his or her teacher. We may underestimate the importance of affect in school learning; drill without appetite, rote tasks, and emphasis on the objective facts can stultify the wide-ranging curiosity of school-age children.

Take for instance the appetite for reading. Of all the reasons why children learn to read there are two that are outstanding. Children learn to read either (a) because they are curious and would like to know "what happens next," or (b) because they have been conditioned to decipher, to decode the meaning of words out of context. The deciphering is not necessarily accompanied by pleasure. One of the authors remembers a child who at the age of four had learned to "read" whole editorials of the daily paper. Thus he amazed adults by deciphering for instance headlines such as "security council proceeds with all due caution" without however understanding the meaning of either "caution": or "security council" or indeed the word "proceed." The accompanying feeling was clearly one of boredom; Herbert seemed to show off his skill, as a trained animal shows off his balancing act.

Elkind (1981) describes movingly the sort of readers some children became after being taught by the rapid drill and punishment method. They read fluently but in subdued whispers and without the joy of discovery and accomplishment. Contrast them to learners eager to understand the content of a story who also are motivated by wishes to model themselves on the beloved adults in their families and to please those adults and their teachers. These readers are in possession of the *real* skill of reading. Their curiosity is the beginning of the chain reaction of learning.

We all know of children who enter grade school full of the triumphs, enthusiasm, and curiosity that has been nurtured by a good preschool experience. Many children today are faced with a grade-school approach that erodes their self-esteem through repeated experiences with failure, since the school's expectations and the child's approach to learning do not match. The spark to learn is not fanned, but extinguished. Many children are left with an abiding sense of *inferiority,* which Erikson (1950) feels is the danger for the school-age child, in contrast to *industry,* the strength for this period. Sarnoff (1976) points out that the school-age child, if emotional issues of the preschool period have been negotiated successfully, is "calm, educable and pliable" (p. 86). He further notes that school-age children deal with the powerful drives usually more openly manifest in the preschool years through fantasy, symbolic play, and the use of such defenses as repression, sublimation, and reaction-formation. If children cannot use these and other mechanisms, they are not able to learn efficiently. They continue to be flooded with feelings which either drain or divert their energies.

IMPLICATIONS FOR PARENTS, CAREGIVERS AND TEACHERS

The preceding discussion has shown how the organizing and propelling force of affects enhance, enliven or retard, and stultify development at all stages. Since affects only flourish in the context of meaningful human relationships, an awesome responsibility rests with parents, caregivers, and teachers. The following section will present guidelines for adults in dealing with children's affects which are based on the previous discussion.

1. *Recognize the significance of "affective reciprocity" in facilitating affective development.* Emde (1980) speaks of the "affective reciprocity" (p. 109) that occurs between parent and infant. This reciprocity continues through childhood and,

in fact, is an essential ingredient in all human relationships. While the child brings to this reciprocity some prepatterned affective structures (Emde 1980), it is the adult who must respond and model in such a way that the child's emotions can differentiate, deepen, and enhance growth in all areas.

2. *Be sensitive to and learn to read the meaning of babies' signals.* Infants experience and express emotions through total body responses and parents learn quickly the meaning of their babies' signals. "Early infant expressions of interest and disgust and later infant expressions of fearfulness, anger and sadness are read accurately by caregivers as indicating need states and as predictive of certain subsequent infant behavior" (Emde 1980 p. 103). Thus, parents, by learning to read their babies affective states and by responding to them appropriately and accurately, highlight the communicative value of affective expressiveness. Caregivers of infants in group day care must take to heart the infant's need for this "affective reciprocity." It is important for caregivers, too, to learn to read the specific meanings of their charges' affective expressions and to realize just how sensitive the babies are to their caregivers' emotional states. Note the abiding affects Jonah still carries with him from his experiences with his beloved caregiver.

3. *Maintain one's equanimity and self-confidence in the face of toddlers' strong affective response to frustration.* Toddlers with their ambivalent stances challenge parents and caregivers. Many of us who have chosen to work with children have strong needs to be seen as the "good" mother. These needs blur our ability to provide support to the enraged toddler who at times, especially when we impose necessary frustrations, insists that we are not "good" but indeed "very bad." It takes a mature adult with an inner confidence to be able to tolerate the feelings of badness that the child occasionally imparts to us. Some adults, however, react by counterattack ("No, *you* are the bad one!") or by emotional withdrawal. The toddler's tenuous self-esteem cannot tolerate such assaults from beloved adults. The caregivers need to understand the all or nothing nature of toddlers' emotionality as well as to possess a fair amount of self-understanding and self-confidence, in order to respond appropriately and usefully.

4. *Utilize the expanding affective development of pre-*

schoolers in encouraging symbolic play which not only helps organize both affect and cognition, but also aids them in self-understanding. The strong emotionality of the Oedipal preschool child presents further trials as well as delights to parents and teachers. The heightened aggressivity of both boys and girls in preschool years leads to frequent limit testing. Further, the competitiveness with the parent and other meaningful adults of the same sex often results in disparaging remarks and outright defiance. Fortunately, preschoolers also can be genuinely loving, full of lively curiosity and creative play interests, which makes this age group especially rewarding and refreshing. Once again, caregivers need the maturity and sense of self-worth that does not get too badly shaken when preschoolers challenge them. They, in turn, can challenge preschoolers by helping them utilize their affective responsiveness through depthful symbolic play which helps organize both affect and cognition.

5. *Build on school age children's affective strengths while continuing to channel emotionality into positive activities and helping children modulate negative emotions.* Teachers of school-age children must recognize that affects continue to permeate childrens' learning. Teachers and parents can build on the positive emotions that drive the school-age child's wish to please beloved adults, to cooperate with as well as compete with peers who are now exceedingly important, and to satisfy his or her abounding curiosity. They can continue to channel the child's emotionality in ways that utilize the child's capacity for fantasy, symbolization, and sublimation. Further, they need to accept, understand, and help modulate negative emotions that can interfere with the learning process: hatred and distrust of adults; jealousy and envy of more successful peers; fear of the new and strange; and shame and humiliation when one cannot meet teachers', parents' or one's own standards.

SUMMARY

In this century, we have had at least two periods in which an educational philosophy was implemented that took into consideration the "whole" child, where emotions were given equal recognition with cognition. These two periods were the

"Progressive Period" of the 1930's and 1940's which was permeated by John Dewey's philosophy, and the "Protest Period" of the 1960's during which the methodology of the "Open School" and "The British Infant School" were put into practice (Glickman, 1984). The teaching reforms of these periods drew strongly from psychoanalytic theory and clinical data. Currently both preschools and grade schools have returned to a heavy focus on academics. With the resurgence of interest in and information about the affective lives of children, we can hope that what was found to be positive and useful in facilitating children's learning can be rethought and implemented in schools.

The powerful influence of affect on children's development at all stages has been emphasized in this paper, along with guidelines for caregivers in helping children deal constructively with their evolving emotions. The psychoanalytic perspective was utilized, with the suggestion that it has a valuable role in shedding insight into the subtle, but pervasive role of affects in human development.

REFERENCES

Benedek, T. (1938). Adaptation to reality in early infancy. *Psychoanalytic Quarterly, 7,* 200–214.

Emde, R. (1980). Toward the psychoanalytic theory of affect, I & II. In S. Greenspan and G. Pollock (Eds.). *The course of life: Vol. I Infancy and early childhood.* (pp. 63–112). Washington, DC: U.S. Government Printing Office.

Emde, R., Gaensbauer, T., & Harmon, R. (1976). Emotional expression in infancy: A biobehavioral study. *Psychological Issues. 10:*37. New York: International Universities Press.

Elkind, D. (1981). *The hurried child.* Reading, MA: Addison-Wesley.

Erikson, E. H. (1950). *Childhood and society.* New York: Norton.

Field, T., Woodson, R., Greenberg, R. & Cohen, D. (1982). Discrimination and imitation of facial expression by neonates. *Science, 218,* 179–181.

Fraiberg, S. (1959). *The magic years.* New York: Scribner's.

Gaensbauer, T. (1982). The differentiation of discrete affects: A case report. *Psychoanalytic Study of the Child. 37,* 29–66.

Glickman, C. D. (1984). Play in public school settings: A philosophical question. In T. D. Yawkey & A. D. Pelligrini (Eds.) *Child's play: Developmental and applied.* (pp. 255–271). Hillsdale, NJ: Lawrence Erlbaum Associates.

Gould, R. (1972). *Child studies through fantasy.* New York: Quadrangle Books.

Greenspan, S. and Greenspan, N. T. (1985). *First feelings.* New York: Viking Penguin.

Hoffer, W. (1950). Development of the body ego. *Psychoanalytic Study of the Child, 5,* 18–23.

Izard, C. E. (1979). *The maximally discriminative facial movement coding system.* Newark, DE: University of Delaware, Instructional Resource Center.

Kernberg, O. (1978). *Borderline conditions and pathological narcissism.* Fifth printing (5th ed). New York: Jason Aronson.

Kohut, H. (1971). *The analysis of the self.* New York: International University Press.

Lewis, M., & Michalson, L. (1983). *Children's emotions and moods.* New York: Plenum.

Mahler, M. & McDevitt, J. (1980). The separation individuation process and identity formation. In S. Greenspan & G. Polluck (Eds.). *The course of life Vol. 1: Infancy and early childhood.* (pp. 398–406). Washington, DC: U.S. Government Printing Office.

Mahler, M., Pine, F., & Bergman, A. (1975). *The psychological birth of the human infant: Symbiosis and individuation.* New York: Basic Books.

Piers, G. & Singer, M. (1953). *Shame and guilt.* Springfield, IL: Charles Thomas.

Piers, M. (1966). *Growing up with children.* Chicago: Quadrangle Books.

Provence, S., & Lipton, R. C. (1962). *Infants in institutions.* New York: International Universities Press.

Sander, L. (1975). Infants and the care taking environment. In J. Anthony, (Ed.) *Explorations in Child Psychiatry.* (pp. 129–167). New York: Plenum.

Sarnoff, C. (1976). *Latency.* New York: Jason Aronson.

Spitz, R. A. (1983). Hospitalism: An inquiry into the genesis of psychiatric conditions in early childhood. In R. Emde (Ed.), *Rene A. Spitz: Dialogues from infancy.* New York: International Universities Press.

Strayer, J. (1986). Current research in affective development. *Journal of Children in Contemporary Society. 17*(4).

Sutton-Smith, B. (1971). The playful ways of knowing. In G. Engstrom (Ed.) *Play, the child strives toward self-realization.* (pp. 13–25). Washington, DC: National Association for the Education of Young Children.

Tronick, E. Z., Ricks, N., & Cohn, J. F. (1982). Maternal and infant affective exchange: Patterns of adaptation. In T. M. Field and A. Fagel (Eds.) *Emotion and early interaction.* Hillsdale, N.J.: Erlbaum.

White, R. (1968). Motivation reconsidered. The concept of competence. In M. Almy (Ed.) *Early childhood play.* (pp. 1–37). New York: Selected Academic Readings.

RESEARCH IN AFFECTIVE DEVELOPMENT

Current Research in Affective Development

Janet Strayer, PhD

ABSTRACT. This paper comprises a selective review of current research concerning affective development in infants and children. The focus of findings and discussion is on three general and related topics: emotion expression and affective interaction in infancy; socialization and regulation of emotion; and children's comprehension of emotions and empathy with others.

INTRODUCTION

Resurgence of interest in affective development, accompanied by methodological advances in its investigation, has led to renewed exploration of inquiries begun decades ago, as well as to newly provocative research ideas and findings. This report comprises (necessarily) only a selective review of some recent research in affective development from infancy through childhood. Adopting the current functional view of

Janet Strayer, is Associate Professor, Psychology Department, Simon Fraser University, Burnaby, B.C. V5A156 and has been a scholar in Affective Development in the Foundation of Child Development Program for Young Scholars in Social and Affective Development.

emotions as adaptive and as part of the individual's organization of experience (Lewis & Michalson, 1983), selective attention is focussed on topics that include emotion expression and affective interaction in infancy; socialization and regulation of emotion; and children's comprehension of emotions and empathy with others.

EMOTION EXPRESSION AND AFFECTIVE INTERACTION IN INFANCY

Perhaps for no other age group is the recent proliferation of emotion research as much in evidence as it is for infants, as attested by recent volumes on emotion measurement and related developments in infancy (Field & Fogel, 1982; Izard, 1982; Lewis & Michalson, 1983; Plutchik & Kellerman, 1983). Infants provide a unique resource for investigation for both universal or biologically programmed emotion expressions, as well as for the early influence of affective learning and socialization.

Measurement of emotion has historically been a hazardous enterprise on technological and on conceptual grounds. Some findings suggest relationships of physiological measures such as heart rate, electroencephalographic, and electromyographic changes with changes in expressive behaviors (Campos, Emde, Gaensbauer & Henderson, 1975; Schwartz, 1982). However, evidence is equivocal at best regarding the specificity of distinct emotion states in infants or adults. In fact, one view suggests that expressions and physiology are inversely related, with facially expressive individuals showing autonomic hyporesponsivity, and vice versa (Buck, 1975).

Infant Emotion Expression Measurement

In contrast, major strides have been made in the reliable assessment of emotion-specific vocalizations and expressions. Different kinds of intensities of infant cries seem to convey different messages of hunger, pain, or anger (Wolff, 1969). Pleasure and, particularly, distress vocalizations of infants have been analysed by Thompson and Lamb (1983), and Scherer (1982) has developed techniques for analyzing infants' vocal expressions related to different emotional states. As regards facial expressions, the microanalytic systems of both Ekman and Friesen (1978) and of Izard (1979), designed to code anatomical changes resulting from facial muscle movements, have revised most recent timetables concerning age of onset of basic emotion expressions.

Current views on the form and intensity of emotion expression in infancy are based, in part, on bio-evolutionary factors that render emotions functional both for the infant's adaptation to stimuli and as signals to others of the infant's state. No certainty exists concerning how many primary or basic emotions there are: Izard suggests 10 and Plutchik suggests 8, (Lewis and Michalson, 1983). Most of these are considered to be apparent during the first year of life: joy, sadness, fear, anger, disgust, interest (anticipation), and surprise. Certainly, parents attribute such emotions to their infants (Johnson, Emde, Pannabecker, Stenberg & Davis, 1982), with anger perceived by 84% of mothers, sadness by 34%, fear by 58%, surprise by 74%, and joy and interest by 95% and 99%. Such agreement may reflect culture-specific attributions or biological universals in expressive behaviors.

Differential Versus Differentiation Theories

Many emotion researchers support differential emotions theory, maintaining that primary emotion expressions are innate, with distinctive neurological substrata for each (Ekman & Friesen, 1978; Izard, 1982; Plutchik, 1983). Other researchers support differentiation theory, maintaining that emotions are differentiated as a function of maturation and cognitive development from ontogenetically similar routes, beginning with "general excitement" or arousal to all stimulating conditions (Bridges, 1932). Adapting differentiation theory, Sroufe (1979) recently described the ontogeny of human emotions. He traced joy from the endogenous smile at birth to the exogenous smile at three months, to laughter at seven months, elation at 12 months, and pride and love at 36 months. Negative emotions were differentiated from rage as exhibited by newborns when their faces were covered or upon physical restraint. Disappointment appeared at three months, anger at seven months, defiance at 18 months, and guilt at 36 months. Bridges never defined "emotion," nor was it evident why a reaction pattern was termed "distress" or "anger," nor was rationale provided for the emergence sequence noted. As for Sroufe's work, some researchers question why guilt is differentiated from anger or pride from joy (Plutchik, 1983).

In contrast to differentiation theory, differential emotions theory proposes that discrete emotions are based on separate, innate neurological programs and are set to emerge when such emotions become adaptive in life. For example, interest, smiling, startle (fear), and distress are present at birth; whereas anger is shown at 4-6 months, when the infant is able to push or kick away the impeding stimulus (Izard, 1982). As indicated in anatomically based recordings of facial expressions, emotion expressions appear earlier for differential than for differentiation theorists. Although infants may show facial movements corresponding to sadness or contempt, however, the question of whether they are experiencing such emotions remains controversial.

Emotion Expressions and Social Context

Regardless of theoretical persuasion, the shift from endogenous and physical elicitors, smiling or crying, to exogenous and psychosocial elicitors, particularly the advent of the social smile in response to persons (Emde & Harmon, 1972), is an important milestone which indicates some voluntary and social control over expressions. While this is a typical occurrence, individual differences have also been noted. Although little is known about their origins, innate and congenital differences as well as socialization, particularly maternal influences, have been suggested (Thomas & Chess, 1977; Thompson & Lamb, 1983).

Caregiver-Child Interactions

These may be important influences for the early development of emotional responsiveness, since both caregiver and child repeatedly exchange emotional signals and regulate social exchange (Capella, 1981; Stern, 1974). Not only is the caregiver's contingent and appropriate responsiveness to infant cries considered important, but the use of a positive and varied expressive repertoire is thought to foster development of animated responsiveness and emotional coping capacities in children (Thompson & Lamb, 1983). In contrast, faced with mothers who similated depression, infants changed from positive expressions, to looking away from the mother, to negative expressions (Tronick, Ricks & Cohn, 1982). Thus, infants appear to some extent able to regulate their emotions and displays to other.

Processes by which early emotion expressions become adapted to social communication functions have been the subject of interesting recent work. Infant expressive behaviors are responsive to environmental contingencies, may benefit from practice, and may be modified by reinforcement and extinction procedures (Campos, Barrett, Lamb, Goldsmith & Stenberg, 1983). Infants also appear to be sensitive to aspects of mother's emotional state, for example, depression (Tronick et al., 1982). However, the encoding channels children use in emotional detection are not specified, and there is little conclusive evidence that infants can discriminate facial displays in emotionally meaningful ways before six months of age (Charlesworth & Kreutzer, 1973; Caron, Caron & Myers, 1982).

The role that caregivers, typically mothers, play in the socialization of emotions has been the topic examined across two representative research areas: reciprocal affect interactions and social referencing. Using microanalytic facial coding systems, evidence from cross-sectional and longitudinal studies of reciprocal affective interactions (Malatesta & Haviland, 1982; Malatesta, 1985) indicates that emotion expression patterns in the first eight months of life change in ways that appear to be based partly on observational learning and reinforcement contingencies present in dyadic interactions. Specifically, mothers were observed over time to decrease the frequency of negative expressions, and increase the frequency of positive expressions. Furthermore, increases in infants' expressivity and positive emotion displays occurred when mothers showed higher rates of reciprocal facial responses contingent on infants' displays, and whey they modeled these positive affects to infants.

Although adults thus appear to influence infants, the bidirectionality of effects also needs to be noted. Malatesta's longitudinal data suggest, for example, that infants' persistent anger displays "may provoke a disinhibition of anger responses in mothers, especially if unmitigated over time, as may be the case with temperamentally difficult babies" (1985, p. 24), thus suggesting a negative reciprocal-effects cycle.

Social Referencing

The infant is an even more purposive agent in social referencing in which she/he searches for information from a significant other person which will help clarify the emotional meaning of an ambiguous situation (Klinnert, Campos, Sorce, Emde & Svejda, 1983). In an experimental example, infants will typically first check their mother's facial expression to ascertain whether or not to crawl towards her across an apparent, but glass-covered "visual cliff." Infants as young as 8.5 months use social referencing to guide their behaviors. No infants crossed over to the mother when she displayed fear expressions, whereas 75% crossed when she displayed joy or interest. Similarly, infants approached by a stranger in an experimental situation were observed to look back and forth between stranger and mother and to smile and show reduced arousal (i.e., heart rate) when mother smiled and cheerfully greeted the stranger, in contrast to fewer or no smiles and increased arousal when mother displayed a frown and stern voice to the stranger (Feinman & Lewis, 1983; Klinnert et al., 1983). As well, they approached toys and resumed activities more following mother's happy rather than angry or tearful vocalization (Svejda & Campos, 1982).

Thus, social referencing may disambiguate social as well as nonsocial stimuli for infants and help them to organize their affect and cognitions. It should continue to operate throughout the lifespan and continue across different cognitive levels and levels of uncertainty. There should be continued questions of interest concerning, for example, the role of familiar versus unfamiliar persons, peers versus adults as information sources, vocal versus facial cues. In addition, the prevalence and developmental sequelae of habitual misinformation, negative information, or absence of needed information from significant others are topics worth exploring.

The Experience of Emotion

Lastly, although considerable progress has been made regarding emotion expression and its socialization, there is little direct research on early emotion experiences. Differential theories suggest a biological link between facial feedback and conscious experience. Many developmentalists, however, maintain that subjective emotion experiences depend upon cognitive developments, particularly acquisition of self-concept, of self-appraisal in the individual's appreciation of what is felt in certain circumstances, what the individual's goals are, and the obstacles to them (Campos et al., 1983; Lewis & Michalson, 1983). Both social and cognitive factors are thus involved in assessing emotional experience. Socialization and cognitive factors in emotion regulation and comprehension are addressed in the remaining two sections.

SOCIALIZATION AND REGULATION OF EMOTION

The socialization of emotion entails, among other things, how and when to express emotions that are, or are not, experienced, how to regulate emotions in ways that are age and socially appropriate, and how to understand such affect management in others. Early parent-child interactions provide occasions for affect expression regulation, both in terms of which emotions are most reciprocated (positive versus negative emotions) and how they are expressed (facial communication seems preferred over loud grunts or wails). Children's adaptation to the social environment also requires that they learn that certain situations provoke expectations about how people should feel and how to suppress or modify expressions so that they are appropriate to self and social interests.

Gender-Related and Individual Differences

There is evidence in our culture of socialization differences that are sex-linked. Adult attributions to infants' expressions certainly appear so; the same ambiguous distress expressions were labeled as anger or as fear if the infant was thought to be a boy or girl, respectively (Condry & Condry, 1976). The same video tape of an infant was considered more negatively expressive when the infant was labelled a boy than a girl (Haviland, 1977). Socialization effects may also be evident in children's expressive behaviors.

There has been insufficient study of preschoolers' and older children's emotion expressions, whereas recent findings indicate individual and age-related differences in children's responses to affect-laden stimuli (Buck, 1982; Strayer, 1985a, b). Boys appear less spontaneously expressive and less adept at posing expressions (Buck, 1982; Zuckerman & Przewuzman, 1979). Nevertheless, the social value of certain expressions seems well organized by most children; social smiles increase from 2-1/2 to 4-1/2 years of age (Cheyne, 1976) and remain particularly prevalent for females in our culture (Feldman, Jenkins & Popoola, 1979; Saarni, 1980).

Socialization Experiences

Socialization experiences influence emotional responsiveness. Children's responses to affect-induction depending on their previous socialization histories (Masters, Felleman & Barden, 1981). Differences have also been noted in the socioemotional responsiveness characteristic of young children who have experienced abuse or neglect, ranging from depressed or shallow affect, to inconsistent affect, to persistent anger (Gaensbauer & Sands, 1979). From an ethological standpoint, as well, Zivin (1977) found that emotion signals are linked to social status. Children of high status in peers' rankings displayed more appropriate facial expressions in winning and losing social bouts than did low ranking children.

DISPLAY RULES

Spontaneous expressions can be also voluntarily or intentionally regulated based upon socially defined contexts for emotions and emotion display rules. *Display rules,* as *symbolic nonverbal behavior,* involve cognitive processing and reflect experiences and learning about self and social constructs.

The symbolic function of nonverbal behavior is evident in facial expressions and gestures which are organized during conversation to support the verbal flow (Ekman & Friesen, 1969). It is also evident when people are asked to pose emotion expressions, or in our daily social rendering of emotion cues. Children's use of emotion to influence others, not merely to express inner states, has been documented as early as infancy (Capella, 1981). As many parents recognize, youngsters may intensify their cries after falling when they are aware of being observed in contrast to when they believe themselves alone (Blurton Jones, 1967). Similarly, children's "coy" behaviors, which seem to signal approach-avoidance to the interactant, are particularly notable across cultures (Eibl-Eibesfeldt, 1974).

As children acquire and refine information about their own affective experiences, they also learn to take account of how others might respond to their overt displays of these experiences. Thus, the communicative impact of emotions comes under further regulation due to demands for social appropriateness and "face-saving" displays, leading to the voluntary dissociation of emotional experience from its expression or, on occasion, to feeling emotions because one "ought to" in the situation. Such display rules (Ekman et al., 1978) comprise aspects of both self and social regulation, and include forms of affect dissimulation (e.g., substitution or neutralization of emotions).

Age-Related Knowledge of Display Rules

Children's knowledge and use of display rules show developmental progression. According to 6- to 10-year-olds, most reasons for emotion dissimulation are to avoid trouble and preserve self-esteem (Saarni, 1979). There are also increases during these years in children's knowledge of display rules to be applied in different situations, with an increase in age-related complexities in their explanations concerning why emotional behavior should be managed and an increase in their knowledge of cultural as well as individual or familial expectancies concerning emotion display (Saarni, 1979). Also, it has also been suggested (Gnepp & Hess, 1985) that display rules are differently understood depending on their mode of expression (verbal versus facial cues) and their motivation (prosocial versus self-protection). Children from Grades 1, 3, 5, and 10 in this study were asked to predict and explain what story persons would say, and to choose what facial expressions they would display in response to story events. Verbal display was better than facial display as reported by all children, with both improving from Grades 1 to 5. Furthermore, all children understood prosocial display rules (e.g., receiving a disliked gift) better than self-protective display rules (e.g., facing an audience after losing a talent contest). The authors interpret these findings to suggest greater socialization for verbal than nonverbal expression, and for prosocial than self-protective motives. However, the latter would appear to depend on the situations or stories samples; Saarni's (1979) results suggest that self-preservation is more prevalent than prosocial motivation.

Age-Related Use of Display Rules

Children not only know, but show display rules better with age. They improve in ability to produce on demand component actions involved in facial expressions; although posed expressions of fear, sadness, and anger are more difficult than happiness and surprise (Ekman, Roper & Hager, 1980; Odom & Lemond, 1972). Age-related increases are noted also in children's intentional control of facial expressions when they pretend to like or dislike an unpleasant or pleasant drink, respectively (Feldman et al., 1979). Socially motivated displays increase with age, with 10-year-olds found to be more successful than younger children in substituting positive expressions for their negative reactions to receiving an unsuitable toy, and boys more negative (less socially-primed) than girls (Saarni, 1980). Yet, while children improve in abilities to mask or control negative affect, they are still unsuccessful in vocal control (Shennum & Bugental, 1982). Causal factors responsible for such expressive control may include previous social experiences as well as cognitive inferential skills such as role taking (Feldman, White & Lobato, 1982). Similar factors may be responsible for children's decoding of others' display rules.

Decoding Emotion Expressions

As we become more skilled in the social regulation of emotion, our skills at decoding cue conflicts in others' emotional messages is also put to the test. In general, it seems at younger ages that there is less differentiation, therefore less detection of disparity among nonverbal emotion channels. We become more accurate emotion decoders with age, yet we still are more likely to be influenced by facial expression, which is a sensitive but controllable display channel, than by voice or body cues, which are relatively less controllable (DePaulo & Rosenthal, 1982). Whereas preschoolers attend to verbal statements in deciphering mixed messages (e.g., "I'm really happy" said in an angry tone with sad face), children from seven years up to adulthood rely on the face as the preferred channel (Mayhew & Strayer, 1985). Oddly, although younger children may be relatively more accurate in judging vocal than visual cues (Bugental, Kaswan & Love, 1970), the face seems to be the major source of nonverbal emotion information with age (Zuckerman, Blanck, DePaulo & Rosenthal, 1980).

That display rules become effective personal and social regulators is supported by findings that children (and adults) are not particularly good lie detectors (DePaulo & Jordan, 1982). Parents and their grade 1 or grade 5 children rated these children's expressions for deception when children tried to convey that unpleasant slides they viewed were pleasant, or the reverse (Morency & Krauss, 1982). Neither first nor fifth graders were able accurately to detect deception in fifth graders, nor were they able to detect deception in first graders. Adults were somewhat better, and were able to detect first graders' deception, but, like the children, could not detect fifth graders "false positive" deception. Lest we think ourselves dupes to contrived emotion information, however, it may be that more impressive detection skills are evidenced in natural contexts in which situational as well as vocal and verbal cues are available. Furthermore, there may be advantages to not detecting social dissimulation or deception as there are social costs to reading unintended even if accurate, messages (DePaulo & Rosenthal, 1982).

A final question concerns the role of parents in children's acquisition of affect encoding and decoding skills. A direct role was suggested by the infancy literature reviewed. Mothers' encoding ability correlates with their children's decoding (Daly, Abramovitch, Pliner, 1981), and mother-child decoding skills are also related (Morency & Krauss, 1982). While correlational, these findings suggest that parents who are good encoders or decoders may provide clear information and feedback to their children. The role of peers and the wider social network has yet to be explored.

COMPREHENSION OF EMOTIONS AND EMPATHY WITH OTHERS

Affect comprehension, necessarily implicated in topics already reviewed, is here considered in terms of children's emotion labeling, their attributions of emotion-evoking situations, and their empathy to others.

Labeling of Emotions

Although abilities to discriminate emotions precede abilities to label them, children produce labels for laughter and crying as young as two years of age (Zahn-Waxler, Radke-Yarrow & King, 1979). Psycholinguistic research has not extensively examined the acquisition of emotion words, yet one early source of such words is likely to be provided by parents. Over 70% of parents used affect terms when reading a picture book to their 2- to 5-year-olds (Greif, Alvarez & Ulman, 1981). Interestingly, whereas there was no difference in amount of affect terms that mothers used with sons or daughters, fathers used more affect terms with daughters. Possible consequences of such early experiences for children's affective language acquisition merit further study. In fact, very recent reports indicate that most children are able to talk about emotion states in the second year, that mothers and 2- to 3-year-olds converse about feelings (Dunn & Bretherton, 1985), and that young preschoolers' knowledge of emotion language in naturalistic contexts is more sophisticated than is shown in laboratory situations (Ridgeway & Barrows, 1985).

Children's acquisition of emotion labels seems particularly relevant for their identification of their own subjective experiences, as well as for their understanding of and empathy for other's emotions.

Emotion Attribution

In addition to knowing how to label emotion; the contexts that evoke them also seems critical to understanding emotional experiences. In a general sense, the kinds of information preschoolers and adults use to infer the causes of emotional reactions appear similar. Information about people (i.e., their dispositions, values, past experiences) is preferred over normative data (i.e., characteristics of the group to which the person belongs), which is preferred over situational information (Gnepp, Klayman & Trabasso, 1982). Thus, although abilities improve, even preschoolers recognize the salience of personal (subjective) reactions when assessing emotional reactions. However, situational knowledge seems particularly important when persons are unfamiliar.

Children's situational knowledge was shown by findings in which 4- to 13-year-olds demonstrated considerable consensus in choosing the probable emotional responses to vignettes portraying success, failure, nurturance, and other conditions (Barden, Zelko, Duncan & Masters, 1980). In contrast, there were developmental differences when children themselves were asked to provide situational contexts for emotions (Strayer, 1985b). Eight-year-olds' used significantly more interpersonal and achievement contexts, in contrast to material goods or events, when attributing situational emotion elicitors than did preschoolers, indicating a greater emotional salience of such contexts. All children studied, however, knew appropriate situational contexts that evoked happiness, sadness, fear, anger, or surprise in themselves and others.

Children's understanding of emotional experience also changes with age to include knowledge, at about 10 years of age, that situations can evoke several conflicting emotions simultaneously (Harter, 1982). Children are also more likely to note that an overt behavior display may not match one's internal emotional experience (Saarni, 1979). With age, they explain the gradual waning of intense emotions as due to internal processes, rather than to changes in the external situation, and know that different emotions affect the interpretation of events (Harris & Olthof, 1982). Such understanding accords with research findings that individuals encode and remember material that is affectively congruent with their mood (Bower, 1981). There also appear to be affective bases for attributional biases. For example, aggressive boys who are faced with ambiguous cues attribute more hostile intentions to peers than do nonagressive boys (Dodge, 1985).

Empathy and Emotional-Behavioral Responsivity

Finally, understanding and vicariously experiencing others' emotions provide the basis for empathy. Although their cognitive understanding is limited, six-month-olds react with interest and contact behaviors toward crying peers, and older children give instrumental aid or reassurance (Hay, Nash & Pedersen, 1981). Even 1-1/2- to 2-1/2-year-olds are aware of others' distress and attempt help or reparations (Zahn-Waxler et al., 1979). Mothers report that by 14 months of age 65% of infants show empathic concern for their siblings (Dunn & Kendrick, 1982). Such evidence appears to point to the sensitivity of infants and toddlers to others' emotions, either as cues to their own states or for other-directed behaviors. Vicarious or shared experience of emotion also seems evident when toddlers, witnessing affectionate and positive emotional episodes at home, responded with similar initiatives and when witnessing anger responded with distress (Cummings, Zahn-Waxler & Radke-Yarrow, 1981).

It has been proposed that individual differences in emotional responsivity are due in part to child rearing, particularly to emphasis on feelings as important (Zahn-Waxler et al., 1979). Similarly, the affective relationship between child and parent has been cited as another antecedent of empathy (Barnett et al., 1980; Eisenberg-Berg & Mussen, 1978; Feshbach, 1978). A likely interpretation is that children who trust that their own needs will likely be satisfied are more responsive to the feelings and needs of others (Hoffman, 1976). Some confirming evidence is provided by findings that securely attached 15-month-olds were rated at 3-1/2 years as more sympathetic to peers than were their anxiously attached peers (Waters, Wippman & Sroufe, 1979). Not only do preschoolers respond empathically to peers in naturalistic contexts, but children highest in positive affect respond most to others' emotions (Strayer, 1980). Empathic children were also found to have empathic mothers (Strayer, 1983), as well as to report their parents as empathic (Barnett et al., 1980). Further suggested is that caring parents, who allow children exposure to a range of emotional experiences, enhance empathy development (Hoffman, 1982).

Lastly, experimental studies indicate that knowledge of others' emotions, as well as shared vicarious affect or empathy, increases with age (Bryant, 1982; Feshbach, 1978). Both verbal reports and, recently, facial expressions have been used. Across studies, there are significant differences favoring females when the measure involves self-report of feelings in response to viewing others in emotion-evoking situations, but more equivocal findings occur when facial expressions are used (Eisenberg & Lennon, 1983). Socialization of emotional responsiveness may permit or encourage females to acknowledge, particularly in verbal self-report, their feelings in response to others. However, as befits society in general, both sexes appear equally able to engage in both affective role taking in order to comprehend others' emotions, and in prosocial behaviors that may be motivated by affective and cognitive responsiveness to other persons.

SUMMARY

In examining the course of developments from recent research reviewed, there are a number of similar and somewhat contentious issues to be confronted. It seems important to convey that developmental changes in affect expression, control, and comprehension seem best understood in a developmental context that differentially weights the contribution of evolution, maturation of expressive systems, and processes responsible for affect detection and discrimination. Additional factors (Yarrow, 1979) include even more complex learning and memory skills, as well as cognitive and social developments associated with affect-related changes accompanying the child's increasing automony, self-awareness, and social and empathic responsiveness. All of these factors influence affective processing in terms of which stimuli arouse emotions, how this arousal is experienced or interpreted, and what is displayed or behaviorally contingent on such affective experience.

REFERENCES

Barden, R. C., Zelko, F. A., Duncan, S. W., & Masters, J. C. (1980). Children's consensual knowledge about the experiential determinants of emotion. *Journal of Personality and Social Psychology, 39,* 968–976.

Barnett, M. A., King, L. M., Howard, J. A., & Dino, G. A. (1980). Empathy in young children: Relation to parents' empathy, affection, and emphasis on the feelings of others. *Developmental Psychology, 16,* 243–244.

Blurton Jones, N. G. (1967). An ethological study of some aspects of social behavior in children in nursery school. In D. Morris (Ed.), *Primate ethology.* Chicago: Aldine.

Bower, G. H. (1981). Mood and memory. *American Psychologist, 36,* 129–148.

Bridges, K. M. (1932). Emotional development in early infancy. *Child Development, 3,* 324–341.

Bryant, B. (1982). An index of empathy for children and adolescents. *Child Development, 53,* 413–425.

Buck, R. (1975). Nonverbal communication of affect in children. *Journal of Personality and Social Psychology, 31,* 644–653.

Buck, R. (1982). Spontaneous and symbolic nonverbal behavior and the ontogeny of communication. In R. S. Feldman (Ed.), *Development of nonverbal behavior.* New York: Springer-Verlag.

Bugental, D. E., Kaswan, J. W., & Love, L. R. (1970). Perception of verbal and nonverbal channels. *Journal of Personality and Social Psychology, 16,* 647–655.

Campos, J. J., Barrett, K. C., Lamb, M. E., Goldsmith, H. H., & Stenberg C. (1983). Socioemotional development. In P. H. Mussen (Ed.), *Handbook of Child Psychology,* Vol. II. New York: John Wiley & Sons.

Campos, J. J., Emde, R. N. Gaensbauer, T., & Henderson, C. (1975). Cardiac and behavioral interrelationships in the reactions of infants to strangers. *Developmental Psychology, 11,* 589–601.

Capella, J. (1981). Mutual influence in expressive behavior: Adult-adult and infant-adult dyadic interaction. *Psychological Bulletin, 89,* 101–132.

Caron, R. F., Caron, A. J., & Myers, R. S. (1982). Abstraction of invariant face expressions in infancy. *Child Development, 53,* 1008–1015.

Charlesworth, W., & Kreutzer, M. (1973). Facial expressions of infants and children. In P. Ekman (Ed.), *Darwin and facial expression.* New York: Academic Press.

Cheyne, J. (1976). Development of forms and functions of smiling in preschoolers. *Child Development, 47,* 820–823.

Condry, J., & Condry, S. (1976). Sex differences: A study for the eye of the beholder. *Child Development, 47,* 812–819.

Cummings, E. M., Zahn-Waxler, C., & Radke-Yarrow, M. (1981). Young children's responses to expressions of anger and affection by others in the family. *Child Development, 52,* 1274–1282.

Daly, E. M., Abromovitch, R., & Pliner, P. (1981). The relationship between mothers' encoding and their children's decoding of facial expressions of emotion. *Merrill-Palmer Quarterly, 26,* 25–33.

DePaulo, B. M., & Jordan, A. (1982). Age changes in deceiving and detecting deceit. In R. S. Feldman (Ed.), *Development of nonverbal behavior in children.* New York: Springer-Verlag.

DePaulo, B. M., & Rosenthal, R. (1982). Measuring the development of sensitivity to nonverbal communication. In C. E. Izard (Ed.), *Measuring emotions in infants and children.* New York: Cambridge University Press.

Dodge, K. A. (1985). *The affective bases of hostile attributional bases among aggressive children.* Paper presented at the Society for Research in Child Development, Toronto.

Dunn, J., & Bretherton, F. (1985). *Conversations about feelings between mothers and their young children.* Paper presented at the Society for Research in Child Development, Toronto.

Dunn, J., & Kendrick, C. (1982). Interaction between young siblings: Association with the interaction between mother and firstborn child. *Developmental Psychology, 17,* 336–343.

Eisenberg, N., & Lennon, R. (1983). Sex differences in empathy and related capacities. *Psychological Bulletin, 94,* 100–131.

Eisenberg-Berg, N., & Mussen, P. (1978). Empathy and moral development in adolescents. *Developmental Psychology, 14,* 185–186.

Ekman, P., & Friesen, W. V. (1969). The repertoire of nonverbal behavior: Categories, origins, usage and coding. *Semiotica, 1,* 49–98.

Ekman, P., & Friesen, W. V. (1978). *Facial action coding system.* Palo Alto, CA.: Consulting Psychologists Press.

Ekman, P., Friesen, W., & Ellsworth, P. (1972). *Emotion in the human face.* Elmsford, NY.: Pergamon Press.

Ekman, P., Roper, G., & Hager, J. C. (1980). Deliberate facial movement. *Child Development, 51,* 886–891.

Eibl-Eibesfeldt, I. (1974). Love and hate: The natural history of behavior patterns. New York: Schocken Books.

Emde, R., & Harmon, R. (1972). Endogenous and exogenous smiling systems in early infancy. *Jouranl of the American Academy of Child Psychiatry, 11,* 177–200.

Feinman, S., & Lewis, M. (1983). Social referencing and second order effects in ten-month-old infants. *Developmental Psychology, 54,* 878–887.

Feldman, R. S., Jenkins, L., Popoola, O. (1979). Detection of deception in adults and children via facial expression. *Child Development, 450,* 350–355.

Feldman, R. S., White, J. B., & Lobato, D. (1982). Social skills and nonverbal behavior. In R. S. Feldman (Ed.), *Development of nonverbal behavior in children.* New York: Springer-Verlag.

Feshbach, N. D. (1978). Studies of empathic behavior in children. In B. A. Maher (Ed.), *Progress in experimental personality research,* Vol. 8. New York: Academic Press.

Field, T., & Fogel, A. (Eds.) (1982). *Emotion and early interaction.* Hillsdale, N.J.: Erlbaum.

Gaensbauer, T. J., & Sands, K. (1979). Distorted affective communications in abused/neglected infants and their potential impact on caretakers. *Journal of the American Academy of Child Psychiatry, 18,* 236–250.

Gnepp, J., Hess, L. R. (1985). *Children's understanding of verbal and facial display rules.* Paper presented at the Society for Research in Child Development, Toronto.

Gnepp, J., Klayman, J., & Trabasso, T. (1982). A hierarchy of information sources for inferring emotional reactions. *Journal of Experimental Child Psychology, 33,* 111–123.

Greif, E. B., Alvarez, M., & Ulman, K. (1981). *Recognizing emotions in other people: Sex differences in socialization.* Paper presented at the Society for Research in Child Development, Boston.

Harris, P., & Olthof, T. (1982). The child's conception of emotion. In G. Butterworth & P. Light (Eds.), *Social cognition and affect.* Sussex, England: Harvester Press.

Harter, S. (1982). A cognitive-developmental approach to children's understanding of affect and trait labels. In F. C. Serafica (Ed.), *Social-cognitive development in context.* New York: Guilford Press.

Haviland, J. (1977). Sex-related pragmatics in infants. *Journal of Communication, 27,* 80–84.

Hay, D. F., Nash, A., & Pedersen, J. (1981). Responses of six-month-olds in the distress of their peers. *Child Development, 52,* 1071–1075.

Hoffman, M. L. (1976). Empathy, role taking, guilt, and development of altruistic motives. In T. Lickona (Ed.), *Moral development and behavior.* New York: Holt, Rinehart & Winston.

Hoffman, M. L. (1982). The measurement of empathy. In C. E. Izard (Ed.), *Measuring emotions in infants and children.* New York: Cambridge University Press.

Izard, C. E. (1979). *The maximally discriminative facial movement coding system (MAX).* Newark, DE: Instructional Resources Center, University of Delaware.

Izard, C. E. (1982). Measuring emotions in human development. In C. E. Izard (Ed.), *Measuring emotions in infants and children.* New York: Cambridge University Press.

Johnson, W. F., Emde, R. N., Pannabecker, B. W., Stenberg, C., & Davis, M. (1982). Maternal perception of infant emotion from birth through 18 months. *Infant Behavior and Development, 51,* 313–322.

Klinnert, M., Campos, J. J., Sorce, J., Emde, R. N., & Svejda, M. (1983). Emotions as behavior regulators: Social referencing in infancy. In R. Plutchik & H. Kellerman (Eds.), *Emotions in early development,* Vol. 2. New York: Academic Press.

Lewis, M., & Michalson, L. (1983). *Children's emotions and moods.* New York: Plenum Press.

Malatesta, C. Z. (1985). *Facial expressions of infants and mothers during early interaction.* Paper presented at the Society for Research in Child Development, Toronto.

Malatesta, C. Z., & Haviland, J. M. (1982). Learning display rules: The socialization of emotion expression in infancy. *Child Development, 53,* 991–1003.

Masters, J. C., Felleman, E. S., & Barden, R. C. (1981). Experimental studies of affective states in children. In B. Lahey & A. E. Kazden (Eds.), *Advances in clinical child psychology.* New York: Guilford.

Mayhew, J., & Strayer, J. (1985). *Age-related differences in decoding discrepant emotional messages.* Paper presented at the American Psychological Association, Los Angeles.

Morency, N. L., & Krauss, R. M. (1982). Children's nonverbal encoding and decoding of affect. In R. S. Feldman (Ed.), *Development of nonverbal behavior in children.* New York: Springer-Verlag.

Odom, K., & Lemond, C. (1972). Developmental differences in the perception and production of facial expressions. *Child Development, 43,* 359–369.

Plutchik, R. (1983). Emotions in early development: A psychoevolutionary approach. In R. Plutchik & H. Kellerman (Eds.), *Emotion: Theory, research, and experience, Vol. 2: Emotions in early development.* New York: Academic Press.

Plutchik, R., & Kellerman, H. (1983). *Emotion: Theory, research, and experience, Vol. 2: Emotions in early development.* New York: Academic Press.

Ridgeway, D., & Barrows, D. (1985). *Young childrens' knowledge and use of emotion language.* Paper presented at the Society for Research in Child Development, Toronto.

Saarni, C. (1979). Children's understanding of display rules for expressive behavior. *Developmental Psychology, 15,* 424–429.

Saarni, C. (1980). *Observing children's use of display rules: Age and sex differences.* Paper presented at the American Psychological Association, Montreal.

Scherer, K. R. (1982). The assessment of vocal expressions in infants and children. In C. E. Izard (Ed.), *Measuring emotions in infants and children.* New York: Cambridge University Press.

Schwartz, G. E. (1982). Psychophysiological patterning and emotion revisited: A systemic perspective. In C. E. Izard (Ed.), *Measuring emotions in infants and children.* New York: Cambridge University Press.

Shennum, W. A., & Bugental, D. B. (1982). The development of control over affective expression in nonverbal behavior. In R. S. Feldman (Ed.), *Development of nonverbal behavior in children.* New York: Springer-Verlag.

Sroufe, L. A. (1979). Socioemotional development. In O. Osofsky (Ed.), *Handbook of infant development.* New York: Wiley.

Stern, D. (1974). The goal and structure of mother-infant play. *Journal of the American Academy of Child Psychiatry, 13,* 402–421.

Strayer, J. (1980). A naturalistic study of empathic behaviors and their relation to affective states and perspective-taking skills in preschool children. *Child Development, 51,* 815–822.

Strayer, J. (1983). *Emotional and cognitive components of childrens empathy.* Paper presented to the Society for Research in Child Development, Detroit.

Strayer, J. (1985a). *Developmental changes in nonverbal expression.* Paper presented at the Society for Research in Child Development, Toronto.

Strayer, J. (1985b). *Childrens' knowledge of the situational determinants of emotion.* Paper presented at the Canadian Psychological Association, Halifax.

Svejda, M., & Campos, J. (1982, March). *The mother's voice as a regulator of infant's behavior.* Paper presented at International Conference on Infant Studies. Austin, Texas.

Thomas, A., & Chess, S. (1977). *Temperament and development.* New York: Brunner/Mazel.

Thompson, R. A., & Lamb, M. E. (1983). Individual differences in socioemotional development. In R. Plutchik & H. Kellerman (Eds.), *Emotion: Theory research, and experience, Vol. 2: Emotions in early development.* New York: Academic Press.

Tronick, E. Z., Ricks, M., & Cohn, J. F. (1982). Maternal and infant affective exchange: Patterns of adaptation. In T. M. Field & A. Fogel (Eds.), *Emotion and early interaction.* Hillsdale, N.J.: Erlbaum.

Waters, E., Wippman, &., & Sroufe, L. A. (1979). Attachment, positive affect, and competence in the peer group: Two studies in construct validation. *Child Development, 50,* 821–829.

Wolff, P. H. (1969). The natural history of crying and other vocalizations in early infancy. In B. Foss (Ed.), *Determinants of infant behavior* (Vol. 4). New York: Wiley.

Yarrow, L. J. (1979). Emotional development. *American Psychologist, 34,* 951–957.

Zahn-Waxler, C., Radke-Yarrow, M., & King, R. A. (1979). Child rearing and children's prosocial intitiations toward victims of distress. *Child Development, 50,* 319–330.

Zivin, G. (1977). On becoming subtle: Age and social rank changes in the use of a facial gesture. *Child Development, 48,* 1314–1321.

Zuckerman, M., Blanck, P. D., DePaulo, B. M., & Rosenthal, R. (1980). Developmental changes in decoding discrepant and nondiscrepant cues. *Developmental Psychology, 3,* 220–228.

Zuckerman, M., & Przewuzman, S. (1979). Decoding and encoding facial expressions in preschool-age children. *Environmental Psychology and Nonverbal Behavior, 3,* 147–163.

Emotional Development of Children With Handicaps

Gilbert M. Foley, EdD

ABSTRACT. This paper examines the emotional development of children with handicaps in the framework of attachment-separation-individuation theory. A modified overview of the normal progression of attachment-separation-individuation is presented in light of current research. Descriptive data on 17 mother-infant dyads followed clinically for 24 months suggests that children with handicaps are at a greater risk for disordered patterns of interaction, delayed progression through the stages of attachment-separation-individuation and incomplete internalization of object and self constancy. Specific interactional risk factors are identified and patterns of attachment-separation-individuation described. An assessment scale is reviewed and a model of intervention for clinical practice is presented.

THEORETICAL FRAME OF REFERENCE

The attainment of object and self constancy stands as a central theme in the emotional development of young children. These constructs refer to the child's internalization of stable mental representations of self and mother as separate people invested with deep feelings (Mahler, Pine & Bergman, 1975).

A remarkable romance unfolds within the first three years

Gilbert M. Foley is Director of the Family Centered Resource Project, Albright College, P.O. Box 516, Reading, PA 19603, and Visiting Clinical Instructor of Pediatrics at the Medical College of Pennsylvania, Philadelphia, PA. A portion of this paper was made possible by an HCEEP Grant (No. G008301514). Earlier versions of it have been presented at the Roundhouse Conference on Developmental Disabilities, The Yale Child Study Center Infancy Seminar, and the Conference of the National Center for Clinical Infant Studies.

of life which lays the foundations for object and self constancy. Mother and infant fall in love, become psychologically interdependent and emerge to negotiate related yet differentiated selves. This first falling-in-love phenomenon provides an interactive apprenticeship for emotional expression and differentiation. Through a psychological process of binding, loosening and identification, the child is born into psychological selfhood.

Margaret Mahler (1968, 1972, 1974) has mapped this journey in a theoretical stage and phase specific progression referred to as attachment-separation-individuation (A-S-I). A modified version of this progression formulated by this author and Sally Provence, MD is presented in Figure 1. It outlines the expected reciprocal themes at each phase and subphase. It is within this theoretical framework that this author followed the course of emotional development in a population of young children with handicaps.

In this paper, reference is made primarily to mothers and children since they were the dyads observed and served. However, much of the data has relevance to fathers and the broader concept of parenting. Thoughtful interchanges, therefore, of the terms mother-child, parent-child and parents and child are made throughout.

The progression of "normal" attachment-separation-individuation occurs in a bidirectional, interactive relationship implying that the partners in the parent-child system effect each other (Osofsky & Connors, 1979). The personality of the mother is central and defines her receptivity, sensitivity and adaptive capacity to serve as caretaker and partner in affective interchanges with the child. The temperament, endowment and sensorimotor competence of the child defines his capacity to elicit maternal responses and utilize mother's availability. The amount and quality of maternal-infant interaction define the opportunity for involvement.

The existence of a handicapping condition in the child has been found to impair the normal development of attachment. Numerous studies have examined this relationship (Blacher, 1984; Blacher, 1983; Foley, 1981; Nix, 1980; Stone & Chesney, 1979), but few have examined the impact of a handicapping condition on the broader construct of attachment-separation-individuation. This clinical study is an initial

ATTACHMENT

NAIVE SYNCHRONY (0-1m)

Child—This subphase of Attachment is characterized by innately provided sensorimotor patterns of action and reaction, tension regulating processes and orienting reflex mechanisms. These behaviors have adaptive meaning and signalling significance which evoke maternal proximity, ministration, empathy and interactional synchrony. The infant's psychological differentiation is rudimentary with no distinction between self, mother, space or time.

Parent—This subphase of Attachment is characterized by a "getting-acquainted-ritual" with the newborn and caregiving which is highly available and responsive. Mother actively familiarizes herself with the newborn's temperament, rhythms and innate patterns of action and reaction. She experiments with styles of holding, feeding, regulating, comforting and stimulating. A seemingly natural and synchronized rhythm of interaction emerges.

PATTERNED SYNCHRONY (1-2m)

Child—This subphase of Attachment is characterized by an expanding capacity for the infant to actively respond to mother and be engaged in pleasurable sequences of interaction. The increasing organization and rhythmicity of the infant's automatic actions and the emergence of more volitional sensorimotor schemes such as social smiling, facilitate the development of patterned interchange. Through a myriad of exchanges the infant slowly acquires a differential awareness between internal and external sources of stimulation and comfort.

Parent—This subphase of Attachment is characterized by active engagement and eliciting of the infant's response capabilities by mother. She employs multisensorimotor means of stimulation, taking her lead from the child and fitting her behavior into the infant's cycles of activity and inactivity. Thus she creates organized sequences of pleasurable interaction and becomes increasingly adept at reading her infant's cues. She can now characterize her infant and has established effective means for meeting the infant's biological, comfort, regulatory and stimulus needs.

SYMBIOSIS (3-5m)

Child—This subphase of Attachment is characterized by sociobiological interdependence between mother and child expressed in empathic mutual cueing—true sensorimotor and affective reciprocity. The child's sensorimotor schemes assume a more volitional and active quality. Affects become more differentiated and discernable and there is a growing capacity to anticipate gratification. While self and object remain undifferentiated there are behavioral indications of memory and anticipation associated with comforting mother-child interaction.

Parent—This subphase of Attachment is characterized by interactive mutuality and affective goodness-of-fit between mother and child. Mother has become very adept at reading and responding to her infant's biologic, sensorimotor, interactive and affective cues. She takes unique pleasure in their closeness, establishes stable patterns of experience, anticipates her child's responses, sets up contigencies and plays sensorimotor games.

SEPARATION

DIFFERENTIATION (5-10m)

Child—This subphase of separation-individuation is characterized by "hatching" from the symbiotic duality and emergent demarcation of mother, self, and other. This is signaled by the preferential smile, sensory discrimination of mother's body, reaction to strangers and comparative scanning. Growing sensorimotor competence contributes to reduced bodily dependence, tentative moving away, experimentation with distal modes of signalling and increased interest in the outside world.

Parent—This subphase of separation-individuation is characterized by the denoument of the symbiotic tie and mother's recognition and support of the child's emerging sensorimotor competence and pull to separateness. She delights in the child's recognition of her uniqueness but supports his signals for flight from the embrace. She assists in his transition from lap-to-floor and supports his turn to the world, albeit with some disappointment. She capitalizes on his alertness by introducing objects into play, providing language stimulation and relating to the child as a social participant. She remains actively and emotionally available and comforts the child in his reaction to strangers.

PRACTICING (10-15m)

Child—This subphase of separation-individuation is characterized by active leave-taking and reunion with mother by locomotor means. The child is infatuated with the world and taken to exploratory ventures. Through these excursions the child rehearses independence, bodily mastery including upright locomotion, distal communication including language and builds an enlarged memory bank of mother. The dominant affect is elation.

Parent—This subphase of separation-individuation is characterized by mother's active but nonintrusive availability to the child as home base and emotional refueling station in his locomotor exploration of the world. She renounces possession of the child's body and offers a gentle push toward independence. She prepares a stimulating environment for him and promotes self-sufficiency. she increasingly uses language to reward, admonish and instruct. She takes delight in his emerging competence and independence, bravado and capacity for affection.

RAPPROCHEMENT (15-24m)

Child—This subphase of separation-individuation is characterized by a renewed need for mother, a now separate person and a beckoning for her love. The child also increasingly realizes his own separateness and with it, vulnerability. This dawning precipitates a crisis characterized by ambitendencies and emotional lability. The child struggles with the wish to restore his "omnipotence" through reunion on the one hand and crystalize his automony on the other. He emerges ,with a more realistic sense of personal boundaries, power and limitation.

Parent—This subphase of separation-individuation is characterized by renegotiation of closeness and separateness. Mother may be confused by the child's return to wooing, ambivalence and restlessness, but remains "quietly available" to him. She is predictably involved, graciously accepts his offerings and responds as a playful participant. She shares in his exploits and offers encouragement toward independence. She increasingly stimulates through symbolic means, supports coping strategies, sets limits and responds with a wider and more complex array of emotions. Conflicts may arise between her interests and the demands of the child.

INDIVIDUATION

BEGINNING OBJECT AND SELF-CONSTANCY (24-36m+)

Child—This final phase is characterized by the seminal attainment of separate personhood. This milestone is based on the formation of two intraphysic structures organized through the progression of A-S-I. Emotional object constancy implies a stable internalized-maternal representation which can be recalled in mother's absence; is invested with positive affect and represents mother as a separate individual with both positive and negative attributes. Self-constancy implies a distinct internal representation of the individual as separate from mother and the outside world.

Parent—This phase is characterized by mother's recognition of the child as an individual and junior member of the family. Mother is able to pursue her own interests and take-leave, with confidence in the child's ability to function well in her absence. She interacts, supports, sets limits and expands the child's emotional-cognitive world through symbolic play and language experiences. She participates and takes delight in the more mature give-and-take nature of their relationship. Mother provides opportunities for the child to interact in the larger world of peers and adults and introduces the child to the challenges of the preschool years.

© Foley and Provence, 1985

Figure 1. ATTACHMENT-SEPARATION-INDIVIDUATION: A DEVELOPMENTAL OVERVIEW.

attempt to characterize the patterns of A-S-I in children with handicaps, identify interactional risk factors created by the presence of a handicapping condition and formulate implications for intervention.

SAMPLE AND METHOD

Seventeen mother-infant dyads were followed longitudinally for 24 months. The average entry age of the children was 20 months with a range between one and 31 months. Eleven children were male and six female. Fourteen were caucasian and two black. All the children were enrolled in the Family Centered Resource Project, a model/demonstration intervention program. Seventy percent of the children were diagnosed as having cerebral palsy and being at high risk for mental retardation. The remaining thirty percent exhibited neuromotor and cognitive deficits of a lesser magnitude and were considered diagnostically as developmentally delayed. All but two children resided in an intact family. None of the families' members had a psychological diagnosis and all provided an average expected environment.

The method of the study was clinical and qualitative. Observations of mother-child interaction were made during weekly home visits by a certified early childhood special educator and during bimonthly casework sessions conducted by a clinical social worker. Data was systematically recorded on the experimental version of the Attachment-Separation-Individuation (A-S-I) Scale (Foley, Mosey & McCrae, 1979) and analyzed clinically for patterns, themes and sequence.

DISCUSSION OF FINDINGS

The results of the study suggest that the presence of a specific handicapping condition in a child increases the risk that normal mother-child interactions will be imperiled and the expected rate and quality of the attachment-separation-individuation process altered. This is not to imply, however, that disorders of attachment and separation arises only from factors in the child. Personality and emotional conflicts of both parents contribute interactively and in some cases can be the primary source of pathogenesis.

The presence of a specific handicapping condition appears to compromise the child's capacity to participate fully in the range of typical mother-child interactions, even in the presence of a competent mother. Children with handicaps are more likely to be deficient in those behaviors which promote and sustain interaction and reciprocity. From mother's perspective this situation might be likened to efforts at stimulating a conversation with a reticent and ambiguous partner or rehearsing a dialogue with a partner who has not yet mastered his lines.

In this circumstance, even if the quantity of stimulation is maintained, the quality may be reduced because sender and receiver are out of alignment and stimulus messages and responses are more likely to be distorted or miss their target. As a result, a qualitative, if not quantitative form of "invisible" deprivation may result. This state is referred to as interactional disparity or dyssynchrony.

Interactional Risk Factors

The following five child-centered factors appeared to be clinically significant in disrupting typical mother-child interactions in the dyads observed. These are: (1) reduced or altered cueing capability, (2) delayed locomotion, (3) disturbances of state and temperament, (4) high incidence of illness, and (5) general developmental delay.

Reduced or Altered Cueing Capability

The normal newborn has patterns of action and reaction that serve as a powerful pre-verbal communicative system. This "language" includes such behaviors as changes in posture and muscle tone, facial expression, rhythmical movements and visual regard. These behaviors promote maternal proximity, empathy and ministration. Mothers look to these cues to guide them in initiating, modulating, altering and terminating interactions.

In the population of handicapped children observed, these signals were sometimes absent, subtle, exaggerated, ambiguous or idiosyncratic. Without clear signals from the infant, mothers were deprived of an important guidance system. They expressed feelings of confusion and anxiety which often resulted in withdrawal from interaction or inappropriate interaction.

For example, one mother asked how she could cuddle and fall in love with a baby who "felt like a board." Another parent, whose child was so hypotonic that her face appeared expressionless, feared her child had no emotions and resorted to pinching and tickling to stimulate a response.

Delayed Locomotion

Self produced locomotion is important in initiating separation. It is a potent signal to the mother to resolve the symbiotic tie, renounce possession of the child's body and revise her perception of the child from infant to toddler. With the advent of locomotion, infants show marked increases in differentiated affective communication and use of mother's emotional responses (Bertenthal, Campos & Barrett, 1983).

The infants followed in the study tended to be significantly delayed in locomotion because of motor deficits. They stayed close to mother, were delayed in making the shift to distal cueing and were more passive. Even infants ready to separate from the standpoint of cognitive and communicative development tended to be kept in a symbiotic stance, because mothers read their immobility as a sign of helplessness. Delayed motor skills tend to inhibit "hatching" from the symbiotic duality. Delayed locomotion, inhibits the normal progression to, and mastery within the practicing subphase.

Disturbances of State and Temperament

Interactional patterns were also stressed because children in the sample tended to be unpredictable or arhythmical in biological needs or bodily functions. Irritability, inconsolability, crying through the night, all presented management problems. Some children had long periods of sleep-like states rendering them unavailable for maternal involvement. These factors tended to test parental limits, precipitate family discord, reduce interactive synchrony with the child and increase withdrawal tendencies. Robson and Moss (1970), also found that prolonged crying, fussing, and demands for physiological caregiving in the infant decreases attachment behavior in the mother.

High Incidence of Illness

Children in this sample and many high-risk infants are more susceptible to illness than normal infants. This frequently results in separation from the mother during critical attachment-sensitive periods. Parents may over-invest or inhibit affectional investment in the child as a stress inoculation against a real or fantasized imminence of death.

General Developmental Delay

Because of a general developmental delay in the observed population, dissonance between maternal estimates of their children's functional level, and the actual abilities of their children were not uncommon. This tended to result in interactions that were developmentally dyssynchronous. This describes maternal interactions which lagged behind or raced ahead of the developmental level of the child. An example of this disparity was observed in mothers who gave up adaptive forms of communication too soon—such as talking in falsetto, gesturing and over-simplified speech.

Patterns of Attachment-Separation-Individuation

The following three patterns of attachment-separation-individuation were identified in the observed population: (1) prolonged helplessness and mechanical mothering, (2) delayed separation and maternal ambivalence, and (3) incomplete internalization of self and object constancy.

Prolonged Helplessness and Mechanical Mothering

The attachment phase in the handicapped population was characterized by an initial honeymoon period motivated by the parent's elation that the child had survived. When the child, however, could not produce synchronous and sufficient feedback to sustain the interactive pitch, a regressive period ensued. A slow and sometimes precarious progression through the subphases followed (Blake, Steward & Turcan, 1975; Kaplan & Mason, 1969).

The tolerance and adaptiveness of mothers for this extended period of helplessness varied. While some mothers delighted in the prolonged dependence of their children, most tended to feel deprived of reciprocal emotional supplies and constricted by the prolonged caregiving. This tended to lead to a strained attachment, a closeness out of necessity rather than fervor.

The interactional style tended to drift into mechanical mothering, interaction with reserve and estrangement. It was characterized by passive proximity and progressively shorter periods of interaction. Maternal ministration and play attempts tended to become more singular, stereotyped and lacking in elaboration. Feeding and diapering tended to become more functional rather than opportunities for affective interchange. One mother said, "I feel like my child is a doll and I'm playing house." This pattern of mechanical mothering suggests that the helplessness of the human infant evokes maternal empathy but the competence of the human infant is critical in sustaining maternal empathy.

Delayed Separation and Maternal Ambivalence

Separation was significantly delayed in the handicapped population, and in part related to the late onset of locomotion. However, when the children began to send motoric separation signals, they were often met with ambivalence on the part of mothers. This was expressed by: (1) difficulty in modulating proximal-distal position to the child, (2) anxiety accepting the typical knocks and falls of motor practice, and (3) poor regulation of their own rescue responses. One mother "sabotaged" her child's practicing efforts every time he crawled away by calling out, "fix your legs," and then hovering close to implement the physical therapy prescription to the letter of the law.

Mothers became accustomed to having relatively helpless children. They had established caregiving routines. When self-sufficiency began to stir in their children it meant "shifting gears" which was difficult for many. Several mothers said, "I know I should help him dress, but it's easier to just do it myself."

The typical patterns of leave taking, exploiting the environment, refueling and reunion which characterize the practicing subphase, were acutely altered by delayed locomotion and maternal ambivalence. This seemed to set off an added cycle of adversity and deprivation in the children, resulting in less efficient desensitization from total dependence on "mother-in-the-flesh" as well as reduced practice in distal signaling, language exchange, use of evocative memory and the development of mediating inhibitory mechanisms.

Incomplete Internalization of Self and Object Constancy

Attachment-separation-individuation is not an isolated line of development. Its progression is tied to motor and cognitive functions. The attainment of object and self constancy was also observed to correlate with representational intelligence, particularly object permanence. This relationship seems to correspond to Piaget's (1981) notion of cognition and affect as two sides of the same coin.

At a chronological age when typical children exhibit readiness for separation, the children in this study continued to need more contact comfort and sensory refueling from mother. They were less able to self comfort and recover from small hurts through the use of memory, play or language. Their affects tended to be less differentiated and more concrete.

The observational data suggest that motor and cognitive deficits associated with children's disabilities: (1) increase the risk for interactional dyssynchrony, (2) contribute to a reduced rate but not altered sequence of A-S-I, and (3) may result in a reduced quality of attachment and a level of object and self constancy which correlates with representational intelligence in general. An increased risk for borderline personality organization also appears to exist. Further investigation of this relationship is warranted. Specific conflicts related to the rapprochement subphase will not be reviewed in this paper.

ASSESSMENT AND INTERVENTION

Assessment

The revised Attachment-Separation-Individuation (A-S-I) Scale (Foley & Hobin, 1981) is an observational instrument refined over the course of the clinical study. It is designed to be used by early intervention providers to: (1) assess the level of

A-S-I functioning in parent and child; (2) identify interactional disparity between parent and child; and (3) identify specific areas of strength and weakness in parent-child interaction.

The scale consists of 168 criterion referenced observational items, reciprocal for parent and child. Items on the parent and child score sheets are organized on two seven level, age referenced continua which operationally define the normal progression of A-S-I. Items are classified into four subscales or domains (sensory cueing, contact, state regulation and discrimination) which appear to be critical substrates in supporting normal A-S-I. The stages and age norms are based on Mahler, Pine and Bergman's (1975) longitudinal sample. Content validity was established by literature and expert review. An interrater reliability study has been completed and a concurrent validity measure against expert clinical judgment is in process.

The scale is scored from naturalistic observations of parent-child interactions and yields full scale and subscale scores for parent and child. These translate into levels of A-S-I functioning and a profile of strengths and weaknesses. Differences in the level of functioning between parent and child (discrepancy scores) are used to identify patterns and specific areas of interactional disparity or breakdown. The profiles provide a basis for developing intervention strategies and tracking change over time.

Intervention

Early intervention for children with handicaps has emphasized the attainment of motor, language and cognitive skills, but the affective aspects of development have been relatively eclipsed. With a goal of comprehensive service delivery, concern for emotional development must be integrated into the comprehensive blueprint of intervention.

The intervention paradigm described here was developed and implemented at the Family Centered Resource Project. It is directed at facilitating attachment-separation-individuation through normalizing parent-child interactions. Emphasis is placed on modifying the handicapped child's cueing capability, promoting the consolidation of development, adapting and amplifying parent's interactional repertoire, facilitating the recognition of the individuality of each relationship, and providing opportunities for ambient play between parent and infant (Korner, 1974; Thompson, Sturm, Proffitt & Morris, 1979).

The following represent broad content areas (Schaffer, 1977) of a "curriculum" for facilitating the progression of A-S-I by normalizing parent-child interactions. They are: (1) cognitive restructuring; (2) normalizing tone, posture and mobility; (3) phasing; (4) adaptation; (5) facilitation; and (6) elaboration. These strategies are intended to be instructional, not psychotherapeutic. This is not to imply, however, that counseling or psychotherapeutic efforts should not be components of a comprehensive early intervention program. The aim of the model is not necessarily to generate new or added intervention activities but to frame activities and experiences already part of the interventionist's repertoire in an affective and interactional context.

Cognitive Restructuring

The goal of this component is to "help parents think more realistically and adaptively about their child" (Blacher, 1984, p. 182). It is important for parents to have information about their handicapped child's condition and level of functioning. Such data provides them with a basis for more accurate reality testing, readjustment of perceptions and expectations, and an explanation for symptoms and confusing behaviors they may observe.

Knowledge imparts a sense of mastery, closes the projective gulf created by the unknown, and promotes accurate identification of the causal sources and meaning of symptoms. Parents need to understand that the extensor thrusting of their spastic cerebral palsied child is not a sign of rejection or the result of some inadequacy on their part. The mother of a difficult-to-feed child needs to know that this problem may be the result of an oral-motor dysfunction and not a lack of some essential maternal capacity to nurture. Parents of a bright, verbal but non-ambulatory child need to understand her strengths and weaknesses to combat overprotection and learned helplessness.

Readjusting perceptions is a slow and arduous process. Patience and repetition needs to be recalled by interventionists. Cognitive approaches in the form of labeling, describing, pointing out features, comparing, contrasting, using analogies and clarifying can be useful techniques in assisting parents toward more accurate reality testing. Ongoing education related to the development of normal and handicapped children can serve as a form of anticipatory guidance.

As the parents' perceptions become more congruent with the reality of their child, interactions tend to become more synchronous, developmentally appropriate and adaptive.

Normalizing Tone, Posture and Mobility

Abnormal tone and posture significantly interfere with normal cueing capability and may misrepresent the true need status of the child. The hyperextended position tends to inhibit a holding and molding response in a caregiver. The flat-bland looking appearance of a hypotonic child tends not to evoke animated playfulness in an adult or peer. The child with a spastic grin is not always smiling.

Normalizing tone and posture is one step toward normalizing reciprocal interaction. As the child's cues become more "readable" and as he feels and responds more as the parents expect, the quantity and quality of interactions are apt to improve.

Teaching parents neurodevelopmental techniques of positioning and handling (Finnie, 1975), not as exercises, but as means to make their child feel more normal and responsive in the activities of daily living, can be very helpful in enhancing interactive pleasure and reciprocity. While the therapeutic positions may seem initially awkward, the improved feedback from the child quickly outweighs the novel motor planning parents are required to master.

In treatment, it is important to ask the mother how she would like her child to feel when she picks him up and what developmentally appropriate responses she would find fun and pleasurable. The physical or occupational therapist might then direct treatment toward experimenting with handling techniques and postures which assist the child's tone and responsiveness conform to parental expectations. The emphasis here is to direct therapeutic efforts toward stability or range of motion as functional means to normalize parent-child interactions as well as enhance postural and motor development.

In the absence of self-produced locomotion, initiation and mastery of separation are likely to be at-risk. If a child shows readiness in the cognitive and communicative areas, but is unable to separate motorically, it is important that some adaptive means of locomotion be considered. Occupational and physical therapists are skilled in finding divergent means for mobility. Scooter boards, hand-operated carts, motorized toys and wheelchairs are a few adapted means of locomotion.

Sometimes therapists are reluctant to facilitate upright locomotion because a child needs more work in prone positions to refine the components of movement. These decisions, however, need to be made in a broad developmental context. There are sensitive periods when one set of developmental needs should take precedence over others. Locomotion and the upright posture are also important signs to parents of their child's growing competence and self-sufficiency.

The author's experience suggests that facilitation of tone, posture, feeding and sensory systems is important in normalizing attachment formation, while the development of motor skills and the facillitation of locomotion are important in normalizing patterns of separation-individuation.

Phasing

Phasing refers to that part of parent-infant interaction that relates to tempo, rhythm and synchrony. The aim of this component of intervention is to assist parents to interpret more accurately the communications of their handicapped children and respond more appropriately in close temporal proximity to their children's messages.

The interventionist acts as a "co-cue reader" with the parents. This can include helping parents to identify more accurately distress, pleasure or state-change signals in their children and establish appropriate contingency responses. It may mean charting the infant's state changes and body rhythms to ascertain a pattern. It may include experimenting with various modalities for altering the child's state, sustaining arousal or providing comfort.

The interventionist's experience with other handicapped

children may help reduce some of the trial and error parents sometimes experience in getting acquainted with their child's unique and often unexpected signals. This component of intervention appears similar to what Umansky and colleagues (1985) refer to as contingency response intervention.

Adaptation

Adaptation refers to the way adults alter their mode of communication to interact effectively with infants and young children, such as talking in falsetto, gesturing and making funny faces. Most parents of children with handicaps do this quite naturally but sometimes get frustrated, give up or move on to a higher developmental level prematurely. Early on, parents tend to follow a chronological time clock of developmental expectations. If the communicative gulf between child and parent widens, it decreases the chances for the attachment-separation to occur.

The role of the infant interventionist is to model and reinforce developmentally appropriate modes of interaction, assisting mother and infant to attain and maintain communicative parity. The experience of the infant interventionist can reassure mother that her infant is on target compared to other infants with similar handicaps, and assist in re-setting her timetable of developmental expectations.

Facilitation

Facilitation refers to the process of bringing the stimulus nurturance of the world to the child through object interactions. Children with handicaps are often poor recipients of such stimulation. Objects presented in typical ways often evade them. For any number of reasons a child may not swipe the mobile, grasp the ring or stack the blocks. Parents may feel a sense of failure or frustration and withdraw.

The role of the interventionist relative to this component is to formulate modified ways in which parents can successfully bring the object world to their child in a spirit of play and pleasure. Too often, activities prescribed for children with handicaps are little more than cognitive procedures or tasks of mechanical conditioning.

In this model, these same activities are placed in the context of social interaction and play. They then function as a means to normalize parent-child interaction as well as cognitive or motor deficits. The emphasis is on mastery of "developmental slices of life" rather than discrete skills.

Stacking blocks for example, can be a developmental opportunity for affective expression, turn taking, inhibition, motor mastery and vocal communication. It can be an opportunity for parent and child to be involved or it can be an exercise practiced over and over until the skill is automatized.

"Activation of the child through play is an essential part of the treatment of delayed or disturbed development" (Provence & Naylor, 1983, p. 51.).

Elaboration

Elaboration refers to the natural expansion of playful interaction that occurs when relating to children. One brings a rattle and suddenly the child tracks it, localizes it, reaches for it. The adult names it, face gazes and smiles, or engages in tactile play. The normal reciprocity and social cues of the infant sustain and transform this singular act of introducing the rattle into a developmental opportunity. A process of "interactive branching" ensues.

Exchanges between handicapped children and parents tend to be more singular, stereotyped and mechanistic. This is largely because the child with a handicap is often limited in ways to signal satisfaction, mastery or provide transitional guidance to the next interaction on a branching scheme. For this reason, the infant interventionist needs to assist parent and child in process-oriented interaction. For example, what to do after dangling the ring. It means formulating chains or progressions of interactive activities rather than singular activities. If elaboration can be facilitated, parents may engage in mutual play more frequently and for longer periods. Greater involvement increases the likelihood for the development of attachment. Elaborated play over time and space is essential in facilitating differentiation of self and affect.

Children with handicaps present parents with a complex challenge. Motor and cognitive deficits can imperil average expected interaction and alter the course of these children's emotional development in terms of attachment-separation-individuation. Intervention needs to expand beyond walking, talking and thinking to include affective development. However, just as one cannot make a person fall in love with another, so attachment-separation-individuation cannot be treated directly. The focus of intervention is to create conditions and opportunities for normalized interaction between parent and handicapped child so that playful and pleasurable involvement will be enhanced and as a result, more typical patterns of attachment-separation-individuation evolve.

REFERENCES

Bertenthal, B., Campos, J., & Barrett, K. (1983). Self produced locomotion: An organizer of emotional, cognitive, and social development in infancy. In R. N. Emde & F. J. Harmon (Eds.), *Continuities and discontinuities in development.* New York: Plenum.

Blacher, J. (1984). Attachment and severely handicapped children: Implications for intervention. *Developmental and Behavioral Pediatrics, 5,* 178–183.

Blacher, J., & Meyers, C. E. (1983). A review of attachment formation and disorder of handicapped children. *American Journal of Mental Deficiency, 87,* 359–371.

Blake, H., Stewart, A., & Turcan, D. (1975). Parents of babies of very low birth weight: Long term follow-up. In Ciba Foundation Symposium 33, *Parent-infant interaction.* Amsterdam: Associated Scientific Publishers.

Finnie, N. R. (1975). *Handling the cerebral palsied child at home.* New York: Duton.

Foley, G. (1981). Attachment and the handicapped child: Development, disorder, intervention. In C. Smith, S. Wimpfheimer & J. Kendall (Eds.), *Reaching out: A resource book for the adoption of children with developmental disabilities* (pp. 255–265). New York: Child Welfare League of America.

Foley, G., & Hobin, M. (1981). *The attachment-separation-individuation (A-S-I) scale* (revised). Reading, PA: Family Centered Resource Project.

Foley, G., Mosey, A., & McCrae, M. (1979). *The attachment-separation-individuation (A-S-I) scale-experimental edition.* Reading, PA: Family Centered Resource Project, Pennsylvania Department of Education.

Kaplan, D., & Mason, E. (1969). Maternal reaction to premature birth viewed as an acute emotional disorder. *American Journal of Orthopsychiatry, 30,* 539.

Korner, A. F., & Thoman, E. B. (1972). The relative efficacy of contact and vestibular-proprioceptive stimulation in soothing neonates. *Child Development, 18,* 95–121.

Mahler, M. S. (1974). Symbiosis and individuation: The psychological birth of the infant. *The Psychoanalytic Study of the Child, 29,* 89–106.

Mahler, M. S. (1972). On the first three subphases of the separation-individuation process. *International Journal of Psychoanalysis, 53,* 333–338.

Mahler, M. (1968). *On human symbiosis and the vicissitudes of individuation.* New York: International Universities Press.

Mahler, M. S., Pine, F., & Bergman, A. (1975). *The psychological birth of the human infant.* New York: Basic Books.

Nix, K. S. (1980). *Maternal attachment behaviors with defective versus normal infants.* (Mother-Infant Studies Monograph). Denton, Texas: College of Nursing, Texas Woman's University.

Osofsky, J. D., & Connors, K. (1979). Mother-infant interaction: An integrated view of a complex system. In J. D. Osofsky (Ed.), *Handbook of infant development* (pp. 519–548). New York: John Wiley.

Piaget, J. (1981). Intelligence and affectivity: Their relationship during child development. Palo Alto, CA: *Annual Reviews.*

Provence, S. & Naylor, G. (1983). *Working with disadvantaged parents and their children.* New Haven: Yale University Press.

Robson, K. S., & Moss, H. A. (1970). Patterns and determinants of maternal attachment. *Journal of Pediatrics, 77,* 976–985.

Schaffer, R. (1977). *Mothering.* Cambridge, Massachusetts: Harvard University Press.

Stone, N., & Chesney, H. (1978). Attachment behavior in handicapped infants. *Journal of the American Association of Mental Deficiency, 16,* 8–12.

Thompson, R. J., Sturm, J. M., Proffitt, G., & Morris, S. M. (1979). Mother-infant interaction and relationship: a review of processes, influences, and effects. *Psychological Documents, 9,* 6. (MS. No. 1806)

Umansky, W., Sanders, W., Baskin, C., & Brooks, D. (1985, Spring). Project explores contingency response as intervention strategy. *Dear Colleague Letter.* (Available from TADS, Suite 500 NCNB Plaza, Chapel Hill, NC 27514.)

Television-Viewing and Family Communication Style as Predictors of Children's Emotional Behavior

Jerome L. Singer, PhD
Dorothy G. Singer, EdD

ABSTRACT. Studies with preschool and early school-age children have examined the links between the patterns of family communication, parental discipline, the children's television-viewing, and their emotional behavior or attitudes. It is proposed that family styles, especially the degree to which parents discuss and interpret the world for children, are important influences on the development of imagination, self-control, and avoidance of unwarranted expression of negative affect or anger. Television-viewing, although a potentially positive influence with limited use and appropriate programming, generally predicts negative affective patterns and aggression. Parent, educator, and clinical approaches to mitigating such negative influences of television are considered.

Children are growing up in a new environment, unknown in human history before the 1950s. It is one in which the formative influences on the child's consciousness, emotions, beliefs, and behavior reflect not only their parents' or siblings' behavior but also the varied and complex input from the television set. Our recent research has been directed at examining the role that parental attitudes and behavior play in filtering the complexity of the world into manageable forms for chil-

---

Jerome L. Singer is Professor of Psychology at Yale University. Dorothy G. Singer is Professor of Psychology at the University of Bridgeport, Connecticut. They co-direct the Yale University Family Television Research and Consultation Center. Address requests for reprints to Drs. Singer at Department of Psychology, Box 11A Yale Station, New Haven, CT 06520.

dren. To what extent do parents also treat the television set as a source of input for children which requires adult mediation? We hypothesize that children's capacities to develop learning skills and self-directed effective use of their naturally developing cognitive capacities as well as emotional control depend upon the extent to which their parents have intervened early and continuously in mediating and shaping the complex environmental stimuli that surround them. With the television set so prominently featured in the American home, watched perhaps four to six hours daily by millions of children between the ages of 4 and 12 (Pearl, Bouthilet & Lazar, 1982), it would follow that parental mediation—or lack of such mediation—of television-viewing may be an important feature of the child's cognitive and affective growth.

DELINEATING INFLUENCES UPON THE DEVELOPING CHILD

Our research strategy has involved first of all identifying the array of potential influences within the home life of the preschool or early elementary-school-aged child which might independently but cumulatively influence the child's emerging knowledge of the world, language and reading skills, beliefs about the relative dangers of the world, imagination, understanding of the television medium, self-restraint or motor control, anger expression and aggressive behavior, as well as behavioral adjustment to school routines. We have examined several different samples of children of lower and lower-middle class socioeconomic status backgrounds. Some of the variables we have measured include two general classes of home influence: (a) the parents' personal self-descriptions or values, their general mediation style, their specific orientation to child-rearing and discipline (including emphasis on physical punishment), and their patterns of daily household organization or recreational activities; (b) the home television environment, (e.g., number and location of television sets, parents' viewing frequencies, children's viewing frequencies and types of programs viewed, and the extent to which parents seek to control and influence the child's amount of viewing, and program selection by imposing rules and by discussing the TV medium.) Space does not permit a review of all the various questionnaire, interview, or home recording devices used to obtain scores for these independent variables. In a number of cases, scores were based on factor analyses of a group of measures. In one of the studies being summarized here, data on parental mediation were obtained not only from parents but from children's descriptions of their parents' behavior in various situations (e.g., during meals, on a visit, at the doctor's office while television was on). Children also reported on whether parents imposed rules about television-viewing.

In effect, then, our home variables may be regarded as encompassing an almost inclusive array of the kinds of influences that may be brought to bear on the child. We have not included measures of older sibling influences because most of our subjects were first born or the older children of their families. Peer group influences are also unstudied, although they undoubtedly are important, particularly with somewhat older children than the 5- to 8-year-olds of these two studies. In general, however, we can regard our home and family variables as reasonably comprehensive potential influences (in addition to presumed constitutional variations) on how the child forms its concepts of the world, learns to use language, to express and experience emotions, to pretend and play imaginatively, and to restrain motor activity or aggressive behavior.

THE SPECIAL ROLE OF TELEVISION-VIEWING

In what special ways may parental attitudes, child-rearing orientations or household-management styles influence the child? There is ample evidence, for example, that children's aggressive behavior (unwarranted physical fighting as distinct from appropriate self-assertion) is linked to familial emphases on violence, frequent physical punishment of children, or the use of power-assertive disciplinary methods (Olweus, 1980; J. L. Singer, 1984). Studies by Tower (1980a, 1980b, 1985) have indicated that parents' own values along three dimensions, *resourcefulness* (imagination, creativity, curiosity), *reliability* (efficiency, competence, punctuality), and *relationship* (friendly, generous, sincere, likeable) are reflected differentially in the spontaneous play or school behavior of children as early as the preschool level.

Of special interest for our research was whether television-viewing patterns of the children might have a special influence over and above these family inputs upon their development. One might, for example, hypothesize that exposure to the varied content and rich vocabulary of television, certainly providing the child with a wider "window on the world" than parental communication could possibly afford, would enhance the child's language use, general information, awareness of "reality", and imaginative resources. Certainly, experimental studies have shown that exposure to appropriate children's programming with some additional adult mediation can enhance positive emotions, cognitive, and prosocial skills such as sharing, friendliness, cooperation (J. L. Singer & D. G. Singer 1976a; D. G. Singer, 1982; Tower, Singer, Singer & Biggs, 1979).

On the other hand, there is the possibility that heavy television-viewing may actually generate an orientation in the child that is counter-productive of the development of useful language, learning skills, and emotional controls. The rapid pacing, intercutting and "attention-gaining by any means" format of television may foster a dependence on direct viewing solely, displacing other necessary self-play or social interactions needed for effective internalization of imagination, practice at moderation and control of emotions and language usage (J. L. Singer & D. G. Singer, 1983a, 1983b). Furthermore, heavy viewing may expose the child to the extensive violent content, car chases, and other grossly active characteristics of the medium and thus impede the building-in of self-restraints or sanction the child's use of aggression as a frequent form for coping with adversity. As the research by Salomon (1983) has suggested, heavy TV-viewing may be associated with a casual, superficial style of cognitive processing, a search for easy entertainment without the attempt to invest the mental effort that would lead to more useful learning. It is possible, however, that where parents take an active mediating stance toward television, and institute rules about viewing or comment about programs, children may acquire a more discriminating and critical stance toward the medium. Children so influenced may fail to show the more negative effects of viewing and perhaps even learn some constructive orientations.

SOME RESEARCH FINDINGS

Let us briefly review some major outcomes of research findings on spontaneous play with normal children. Pairs of observers recorded the behavior and verbalization of preschoolers during "free play" periods. We have now studied more than 300 children through repeated observation. After recording what the children said and did for ten minute periods on eight separate occasions over a year's time, raters scored these transcripts on predefined variables such as *imaginativeness of play, positive affect* or *emotionality* (e.g., smiling, laughing, interest and curiosity), *cooperation with other children,* acts of *aggression,* (D. G. Singer & J. L. Singer, 1980; J. L. Singer & D. G. Singer, 1981). On the basis of factor analyses of the behavior and verbalization patterns we consistently found two or three major dimensions along which the children varied. One dimension is perhaps best labelled as *playfulness*. A child who scored high on the variables that make up this factor shows a good deal of make-believe during play, generally positive emotional expressiveness, and very little evidence of sadness, fear or fatigue. These imaginative children are also more cooperative with other children and are rated high on *leadership*.

A second dimension that emerges regularly, *aggression,* is characterized by evidence of aggressive activity and involvement in fights, the emotion of anger shown more often during observation periods, and, from parent records of the children's home TV-watching (maintained across the year), greater tendency to watch action or violent programming as well as heavier TV-viewing generally. Indeed still a third study across a longer time period showed the link between heavy viewing, especially of more violent programming, aggression, and poor behavioral adjustment in the early school years (J. L. Singer, D. G. Singer & Rapaczynski, 1984a).

A third dimension emerges which shows a positive second-order relationship to *playfulness* and a negative second-order relationship to the *aggression* dimension. This factor reflects evidence of more internalized imagination (e.g., as reflected in imaginary playmates, higher scores on inkblot measures of fantasy) and is reflected in generally more cooperative and adaptive school behavior. Older preschool children and girls tend to score higher on this dimension which can be called *internalized imagination and social maturity* (J. L. Singer & D. G. Singer, 1981).

PARENTAL BEHAVIOR AND TV IN CHILDREN'S COGNITION AND FEARFUL BELIEFS

In discussing our results with respect to parents, we will be condensing findings for two separate investigations, one involving predictions of behavior across several years from the independent variables (J. L. Singer, D G. Singer, Rapaczynski, 1984a, 1984b) and the second, a shorter-term prediction based, on more extensive data collected from children as well as mothers on the parents' behavior (Desmond, et al., 1985; J. L. Singer & D. G. Singer, 1985a). The basic data analysis tactic is that of multiple regression analysis in which we seek to determine what combination of independent variables yields the highest prediction of the child's cognitive and behavioral patterns. This procedure also permits us to estimate whether family or television variables make *independent* conttributions to our prediction equations thus providing evidence on whether television effects may simply reflect general familial orientations (e.g., children from certain families simply like more TV, or whether television-viewing predicts behavior even when other variables are already accounted for).

Our data indicate that the child's early reading readiness/achievement is best predicted by an independent combination of family and television-viewing variables. More specifically, when parents themselves adopt a view of the world as a hostile, "scary" place, when the children watch more television, and when the family is from a lower social class (a smaller effect), children show poor reading scores. For general information, our data yield a generally similar result. While general intelligence as measured by the Peabody Picture Vocabulary Test is the best predictor of the child's general information knowledge, a combination of variables including less television-watching by the child, more television rules imposed by parent (child's report), a less fearful view of the world by parents, and greater parental self-evaluation as imaginative and resourceful, all add substantially and independently to the prediction. Essentially, a similar result emerges for the child's effective use of language.

Turning to fearfulness, as measured by beliefs in a scary world, our data were especially strong in indicating that heavy TV-viewing by the child, especially of the more violent, realistic action-adventure programming is predictive of later beliefs in a more frightening or dangerous immediate environment (J. L. Singer, D. G. Singer & Rapaczynski, 1984a). The child's perception of the mother as more frequently making negative comments about situations plus the failure of parents to impose rules about television-viewing predicted the higher "Scary World" scores in children. In a subsequent study (in preparation), we found that the heavier the general TV-viewing and the less mediation and discussion by parents, the higher the scores were on fears about the world, a year later.

We also considered the ability to discriminate real from fantasy occurrences (e.g., "Can a man stop a speeding train with his hands?"). It was predicted best by the child's intelligence, by the family's imposition of rules about TV-viewing (as reported by the child), by the amount of time spent watching television, by the disciplinary stance taken by parents, and by the amount of time spent explaining television events to the child. In effect, the heavy-viewing child whose parents put few restrictions on viewing and made less effort to mediate the environment was more likely to confuse fantasy and impossible events with reality.

IMAGINATION, PARENTAL INFLUENCE, AND TELEVISION-VIEWING

Let us take a more extended look at the special role of imaginative play in the early affective development. It seems clear that children of at least average intelligence have some inclination towards imaginative play. It helps them organize the complexities of the environment, miniaturize novelty and "big things" like automobiles, airplanes, or even Mommy and Daddy into manageable cognitive proportions (Tomkins, 1970) which can then be assimilated as Piaget (1962) proposed into established schema. The very act of organizing such material, the development of a story-line and the change of the unfamiliar to the familiar through make-believe evokes the positive affects of interest-excitement and joy (J. L. Singer, 1973).

But children usually need some additional adult help to sustain and broaden the scope of their capacity for imaginative play. Here the adult is crucial. Story-telling or reading encourages the child to use its imagery capacities, provides *content* for play plots, and establishes an atmosphere that makes fantasy an acceptable form of childhood activity. The parent who initiates a make-believe game and then steps back once it is underway and permits the child to develop his/her own independent momentum is, in effect, training a child to develop the skills needed for effective spontaneous play (J. L. Singer & D. G. Singer, 1976b; Shmukler, 1981). Viewed from this perspective, fostering imaginative play in children can be seen as a basic inculcation of a major ego function or as a component of the *mediated learning systems* approach emphasized by Feuerstein (1977) in his theory of cognitive modifiability.

The most extensive research evidence now available suggests that children who are heavy viewers of television show less spontaneous fantasy in spontaneous play or in tests of imagination (D. G. Singer, 1982; J. L. Singer and D. G. Singer, 1983b). Quite possibly the ease of obtaining the pleasures of story telling through watching television suffices to displace the necessary practice of this skill through active self-talk, private imagery, manipulation of blocks or toys and cooperation in the structures and sequences of make-believe play with other children (J. L. Singer & D. G. Singer, 1981). Yet under proper conditions exposure to appropriate television programming can stimulate imagination. Studies of the *Mister Rogers' Neighborhood* program with its carefully delineated Neighborhood of Make Believe and of special programming designed in Australia and England indicate that imaginative behavior increases after several weeks of exposure especially if further enhanced by input from an adult

(Friedrich & Stein, 1975; D. G. Singer, 1982; J. L. Singer & D. G. Singer, 1976a; Tower et al., 1979).

We have elsewhere elaborated on research which supports a number of specific cognitive, affective, and social advantages for the growing child of an early development of imaginative play skills. To summarize briefly: children who show make-believe tendencies seem also generally happier, more capable of richer vocabulary and divergent or creative thought, and more able to tolerate delays or to amuse themselves in boring or strange environments. They are also more likely to be more socially cooperative, to make distinctions between reality and fantasy, to be empathic, and less likely to engage in unprovoked acts of aggression. By contrast children and adolescents who show an absence of imaginative or fantasy skills or interests often prove to be more restless, impulsive, aggressive, involved in antisocial acts, and prone to unpleasant moods or emotions (J. L. Singer and D. G. Singer, 1976b; J. L. Singer & Brown 1977).

It would follow from such evidence that we need to pay a good deal more attention in child-rearing to establishing conditions conducive to enhancing the effective use of the child's imaginative potentialities. This approach can take several forms. An important first step is to reach parents and to help them understand that child care involves not only physical nurturance but also basic affection and cognitive skill training. Affection is experienced by the child not only through parents' positive regard but through their concrete acts which foster imaginative play, and through their story-telling and shared make-believe.

Without denying that good parenting may "come naturally" to many young people, experience with many families suggests that some raising of adults' consciousness about the importance of children's play is necessary. In the various research studies we carried out over the last 12 years, we have talked with hundreds of parents and have recognized that many are still uncomfortable or uncertain about how to play with their children and especially how to foster imaginative games. Many parents are still queasy about the possibility that make-believe games and fantasy create an "unrealistic" child. We have had to develop a whole series of exercises through which parents can first of all regain contact with their own childhood. By relaxing and allowing their minds to drift back to their bedrooms at age five, to the toybox they may have had, to a favorite stuffed animal, to first friends, parents soon retrieve a sense of how much they enjoyed make-believe and fantasy as a child or the occasional story-telling of a parent. We have developed a graded series of exercises and games which parents can introduce to preschool children to foster sensitivity to the environment and then to foster an increasing capacity to manipulate symbols, and to play imaginatively (D. G. Singer & J. L. Singer, 1977, 1985). Parents need help to see just how they can play a part in encouraging and initiating imagination and, then, how to back off and let the child carry forward the game under his/her own momentum.

There seems little doubt from research evidence that children respond with excitement to adult leadership in the area of imaginative play. We have shown that other adult caretakers can often stimulate imaginativeness in very young children and create a more enjoyable play atmosphere which the children carry further on their own and will initiate spontaneously later on. Intervention by teachers or researchers through thematic fantasy play with a wide range of preschool and early school age children has been shown in a whole series of studies to yield increased positive affect, empathy, creative behavior, and cooperative or school adaptive attitudes as well as improved cognitive performance (J. L. Singer et al., 1977; D. G. Singer, 1978). We have also explored the possibility that particular television programming designed especially for children will lead to more imaginative play, positive affect and "prosocial" behavior (D. G. Singer, 1978, 1982; D. G. Singer & T. Revenson, 1978; D. G. Singer & J. L. Singer, 1976; J. Singer & D. Singer, 1976a; Tower, Singer, Singer and Biggs, 1979). Research has shown that the TV cannot replace the "live" adult in effectiveness of stimulating imaginative play. Still, a benign program like *Mister Rogers' Neighborhood* with a consistent, caring host who talks softly and slowly and who encourages "pretending" through a careful separation of reality and make-believe sequences, has important positive mental possibilities because of the mass audience for TV. We need many more programs designed for young children that emphasize imagination and the constructive social values of sharing and cooperation. Parents must be involved, too. As our data indicates, the combination of a *less* TV-viewing and a *more* imaginatively oriented parent predicted more creative block-play or imaginative response to inkblots by the children (Singer, Singer & Rapaczynski, 1984b).

UNDERSTANDING TELEVISION PLOTS AND FORMAT

With respect to the child's ability to comprehend and to reproduce clearly the plots of television programming, our data clearly indicate the combined effects of the parental role in the television medium. Children who reported that their parents imposed rules about television-watching, whose mothers themselves watched *less* television, and who described their mothers as likely to make positive remarks in a variety of situations were *better* able to identify plot details or to provide organized accounts of what they'd witnessed in an episode of *Swiss Family Robinson.* These results are independent of the children's intelligence or the family's social class background. When we turn to the child's comprehension of the nature and purpose of commercial advertising on television, the combination of a parental style emphasizing mediation generally as well as one imposing rules on television (child's report) predicts better comprehension along with but independent of the child's IQ and SES background. Family mediation also plays an important role in predicting the child's ability to explain special effects such as "zooms" (Desmond et al., 1985).

RESTLESSNESS, AGGRESSION AND SCHOOL BEHAVIOR

We can turn next to some possible family and television correlates of the overt behavior of the child. We measured restlessness or lack of self-restraint in a number of ways, (e.g., inability to sit still for a long period in a simulated astronaut capsule, restlessness as observed during an observed waiting period of ten minutes, and restlessness and impulsive motor activity while watching some films with a parent). Our results consistently implicate heavy television-viewing by the child, especially of the more violent programming, in predicting greater restlessness or less ability to sit quietly. Factors such as the child's report that the mother is more likely to be pleasant and supportive in various situations, parents who describe themselves as more imaginative and creative, and who run a more orderly household all combine in predicting less restless behavior by the child (Singer, Singer & Rapaczynski, 1984a; Singer & Singer, 1985).

The prediction of overt aggressive behavior in a child shows a generally similar pattern. Heavier viewing of violent programming or of television, heavier viewing of television by parents, and, in general, more overall emphasis by parents on physical discipline and power-assertion all predict greater aggressive behavior by the children. The same results emerge when school reports of poor behavioral adjustment are used as the dependent variables (J. L. Singer, D. G. Singer & Rapaczynski, 1984a).

A rather clear and dramatic indication of how parental communication style and the child's television-viewing combine to predict the child's aggressive behavior one year later can be found in Figure 1, based on data from Singer & Singer (1985a). In this study children were 5 at initial testing; data on children's television-viewing across a year and on the mothers' style of communication or mediation of the environment in various situations (based on mothers' reports) were obtained. A year later, the mothers described in detail their children's responses to a variety of daily life situations and these behaviors were scored for overt, physical aggression. Four groups of children were identified by median splits of the distributions of scores on *Mothers' Discussion vs. Prescription* (Mediation) and *Child's Television-viewing:* (1) High Mediation, Low TV-viewing, (2) High Mediation, High TV-viewing, (3) Low Mediation, Low TV-viewing and (4) Low Mediation, High TV-viewing. As Figure 1 indicates, children who watch little television and whose mothers engage in more general discussion and explanation are the least aggressive a year later; high mediation and high television-viewing predicts more aggression but much less than low mediation and high television-watching, the condition that predicts greatest aggression. Similar results were found for the children's restlessness as observed by objective raters and for the children's scores on fearfulness about the outside world (Singer & Singer, 1985a).

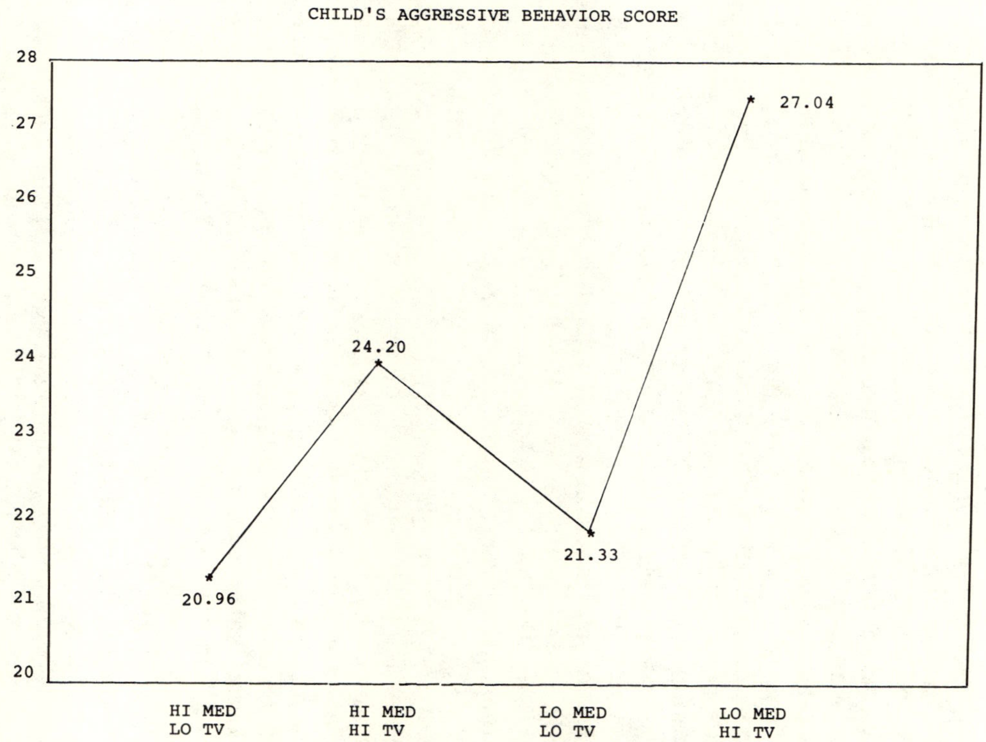

Figure 1: The scores on reported aggressive behavior as a function of children's combined group scores on hours of television-viewing and on the discussion versus prescription factor score.

SOME CONCLUSIONS: PARENTAL CONTROL OF TELEVISION

In summary, our study of family patterns and their relationship to television-viewing and children's development lead to a clear indication of the combined influences of parental styles and television-viewing on the emerging cognitive and behavioral tendencies of elementary school children of both sexes. We have identified several types of family patterns that seem especially relevant to the child's acqusition of cognitive skills and to the child's development of motor restraint, less aggression, and better school behavioral adjustment. These include parents who (1) personally value imagination and resourcefulness or responsibility and stability, (2) do not emphasize power-assertive discipline and physical punishment, (3) actively mediate the outside world for children through explanation and discussion rather than preemptory discipline or judgmental assertions, and (4) watch less television themselves and who hold a less "mean and scary" view of their environment. These family life variables are not sufficient to explain the child's cognitive and behavioral scores. The amount and type of the child's television-viewing does prove to be an important predictor of behavior; indeed, it seems clear from our own studies that heavy TV-viewing puts the child at serious risk by early school age of failing to obtain significant world information, of poor reading skills, of poor discrimination of reality from fantasy, less imaginative skill, of a more fearful view of the world; and of greater restlessness and more aggression, all contributory to poor behavioral adjustment when the child is beginning at school.

A critical role seems to be played, however, by parental intervention in the child's use of television. Thus even without a more general mediating family style, parents who set rules about television-viewing, who prescreen programs from newspaper guides, or who discuss and restrict viewing may indeed be establishing an atmosphere that leads the child towards more critical viewing. We conclude that parents, clinicians, and educators must increasingly recognize that an important feature of child-rearing requires careful attention to the role of the television set in the child's daily life.

Our studies and our work with parent and school groups

suggest several avenues for effective early intervention with children. We have developed a series of eight school lessons for children in the early elementary grades that explain how television works, how special effects are produced, the role of violence and the stereotypes in TV-content, the purpose and potential deceptiveness of commercials, how news is edited (D. G. Singer, J. L. Singer & Zuckerman, 1981). Research studies and application in schools suggest the value of such an approach (D. G. Singer, Zuckerman, & J. L. Singer, 1980; Rapaczynski, D. G. Singer & J. L. Singer, 1982). Special guides for parents and teachers are also available that are designed to alert them to an early establishment of television rules, to increased use of restrictions on frequency and pattern of viewing (e.g., "only *after* school homework") and to discuss constructive content from shared viewing experiences (D. G. Singer & J. L. Singer, 1981; D. G. Singer, J. L. Singer & Zuckerman, 1981). We cannot change over all family structures but we hope to raise parental consciousness so that parents can decide who is to raise their children, the live adults in the home or the fantasy figures on television. Clinicians and educators can also play a crucial role in alerting parents to these issues, in mediating television and in exploring children's expectations, abuse, and misinterpretation of the medium. Television and related forms of visual entertainment (videodiscs and videotapes) are here to stay; specialists in children and family life must adjust their approaches to recognizing this potentially hazardous (if occasionally benevolent) intruder into the bosom of the family.

REFERENCES

Desmond, R. J., Singer, J. L., Singer, D. G., Calam, R., & Colimore, K. (1985). Family mediation patterns and television viewing: Young children's use and grasp of the medium. *Human Communications Research, 11,* 461–80.

Feuerstein, R. (1977). Mediated learning experience: A theoretical basis for cognitive modifiability during adolescence. In P. Mittler (Ed.), *Research to practice in mental retardation: Education and training* (Vol. 2). Baltimore: University Park Press.

Friedrich, L. K., & Stein A. H. (1975). Prosocial television and young children: The effects of verbal labeling and role playing on learning and behavior. *Child Development, 46,* 27–38.

Olweus, D. (1980). Familial and tempermental determinants of aggressive behavior in adolescent boys: A causal analysis. *Developmental Psychology, 16,* 644–60.

Pearl, D., Bouthilet, L., & Lazar, J (Eds.). (1982). *Television and behavior: Ten years of scientific progress and implications for the eighties* (Vol. 2). Washington, DC: U.S. Government Printing Office.

Piaget, J. (1962). *Play, dreams and imitation in childhood.* New York: Norton.

Rapaczynski, W., Singer, D. G., & Singer, J. L. (1982). Teaching television: A curriculum for young children. *Journal of Communication, 32,* 46–55.

Salomon, G. (1983). Television watching and mental effort: A social psychological view. In J. Bryant & D. Anderson (Eds.), *Children's understanding of television.* New York: Academic Press.

Shmukler, D. (1981). Mother-child interaction and its relationship to the predisposition of imaginative play. Genetic Psychology Monographs, 104, 202–25.

Singer, D. G. (1978). Television and imaginative play. *Journal of Mental Imagery, 2,* 145–64.

Singer, D. G. (1982). Television and the developing imagination of the child. In P. Pearl. L. Bouthilet, & J. Lazar (Eds.), *Television and behavior: Ten years of scientific progress and implications for the eighties* (Vol. 2). Washington, DC: U. S. Government Printing Office.

Singer, D. G., & Revenson, T. (1978). *A Piaget primer: How a child thinks.* Bergenfield, N.J.: New American Library.

Singer, D. G., & Singer, J. L. (1976). Family television viewing habits and the spontaneous play of preschool children. *American Journal of Orthopsychiatry, 46,* 446–502.

Singer, D. G., & Singer, J. L. (1977). *Partners in play.* New York: Harper & Row.

Singer, D. G., & Singer, J. L. (1980). Television viewing and agressive behavior in preschool children: A field study. *Annals of the New York Academy of Sciences, 347,* 292–303.

Singer, D. G., & Singer, J. L. (1981). *Getting the most out of television: Videotapes.* Northbrook, IL: MTI Teleprograms.

Singer, D. G., & Singer, J. L. (1985). *Make-believe: Games and activities to foster imaginative play in young children.* Glenview, IL: Scott, Foresman.

Singer, D. G., Zuckerman, D., & Singer, J. L. (1980). Helping elementary school children learn about TV. *Journal of Communication, 30,* 84–93.

Singer, J. L. (1973). *The child's world of make-believe: Experimental studies of imaginative play.* New York: Academic.

Singer, J. L. (1977). Imagination and make-believe play in early childhood: Some educational implications. *Journal of Mental Imagery, 1,* 127–44.

Singer, J. L. (1984). *The human personality.* San Diego: Harcourt, Brace, Jovanovich.

Singer, J. L., & Brown, S. L. (1977). The experience type: Some behavioral correlates and theoretical implications. In M. C. Rickers-Ovsiankina (Ed.), *Rorschach psychology.* New York: Springer.

Singer, J. L., & Singer, D. G. (1976a). Fostering creativity in children: Can TV stimulate imaginative play? *Journal of Communication, 26,* 74–80.

Singer, J. L., & Singer, D. G. (1976b). Imaginative play in early childhood: Some experimental approaches. In A. Davis (Ed.), *Child personality and psychopathology.* New York: Wiley.

Singer, J. L., & Singer, D. G. (1981). *Television, imagination and agression: A study of preschoolers.* Hillsdale, NJ: Erlbaum.

Singer, J. L., & Singer, D. G. (1983a). Implications of childhood television viewing for cognition, imagination and emotion. In J. Bryant & D. Anderson (Eds.), *Children's understanding of television.* New York: Academic Press.

Singer, J. L., & Singer, D. G. (1983b). Psychologists look at televeision: Cognitive developmental and social policy implications. *American Psychologist, 38,* 826–34.

Singer, J. L., & Singer, D. G. (1985). *Television and family living patterns: A study of preschoolers and their parents.* (Progress Report #3 to the MacArthur Foundation).
Singer, J. L., Singer, D. G., & Rapaczynski, W. (1984a). Children's imagination as predicted by family patterns and television viewing: A longitudinal study. *Genetic Psychology Monographs, 110,* 43–69.
Singer, J. L., Singer, D. G., & Rapaczynski, W. (1984b). Family patterns and television-viewing as predictors of children's beliefs and aggression. *Journal of Communication, 34,* 73–89.
Tomkins, S. S. (1970). A theory of memory. In J. Antrobus (Ed.), *Cognition and affect.* Boston: Little, Brown & Co.
Tower, R. B. (1980a). The influence of parents' values on preschool childrens' behavior. Unpublished doctoral dissertation, Yale University, New Haven.
Tower, R. B. (1980b). *Journal of Personality and Social Psychology, 39,* 710–18.
Tower, R. B. (1985). Preschoolers' imaginativeness: Subtypes, correlates, and maladaptive extremes. *Imagination, Cognition and Personality, 4,* 349–364.
Tower, R. B., Singer, D. G., Singer, J. L. & Biggs, A. (1979). Differential effect of television programming on preschooler's cognition, imagination and social play. *American Journal of Orthopsychiatry, 49,* 265–28.

Where Have All the Players Gone?

Nancy E. Curry, PhD

ABSTRACT. This paper examines the relationship of play and language to the development of the sense of self. The value of playful, affectively charged interchanges between caregivers and children is highlighted. This developmental framework gives guidelines to diagnose where children may be on the play continuum. For children who seem developmentally delayed in terms of language and play, an intervention model is proposed which parallels the playful interventions good parents use to enhance the optimal self-devclopment of their children.

INTRODUCTION

For the past two years I have been a member of a mental health consultation team for a local preschool program for disadvantaged 3- and 4-year-olds. Observing the children in their classrooms, conferring with their teachers, and assessing their play skills, the team members have been struck by the relative absence of pretend play and the limited language used by these children. Concomitantly, I have engaged in

Nancy E. Curry is professor and program director of Child Development and Child Care, School of Health Related Professions, University of Pittsburgh. Requests for reprints may be directed to 213 Pennsylvania Hall, School of Health Related Professions, University of Pittsburgh, Pittsburgh, PA 15261.

another consulting enterprise in which I viewed videotapes of low income young mothers and their 1-year-olds. Here, too, it is striking to note the absence of language and play in the interactions between these young mothers and their babies. The zest and vigor of the practicing child and the mood of elation that Mahler and her colleagues (Mahler, Pine & Bergman, 1975) describe so well, are absent in these infant/mother pairs. Much of this has been reported in the literature (e.g., Baldwin & Baldwin, 1973; Hess & Shipman, 1965; Bee, Van Egeren, Streissguth, Nyman, & Leckie, 1969; Schachter, 1979; Snow, Arlman-Rupp, Hassing, Jobse, Joosten & Vorster, 1976). Yet the fact that it continues to exist, in spite of what we have attempted through intervention programs, is unsettling.

Equally unsettling is the fact that the phenomenon of the nonplaying preschooler is not isolated to disadvantaged preschoolers. Child development students report the dearth of depthful, extended pretend play episodes in their practicum placements, often centers with middle-class children. My own observations support theirs. "Free play time" is given token recognition on most teachers' schedules, but appears to be a space filler between what many teachers view as the "important" activities of the day: extended group times in which the children parrot back to their teachers the alphabet, numbers, the days of the week, the month, colors, shapes, and other rote memory tasks; group craft projects in which each child makes the symbol of the current holiday (turkeys, ghosts, rabbits, Christmas trees, and even silhouettes of Lincoln and Washington); the routines of toileting and preparing for meals.

Where have all the players gone? Informal observation of preschoolers of family and friends reveal that they still are busily playing at home and in school settings wherever more than a token recognition is given to the importance of pretend play. While there are undoubtedly many factors responsible for the lack of observable play episodes in many preschool settings, three stand out.

First, there are children who do not seem to have the developmental underpinnings necessary to deal adequately with the symbol sytems of either play or language.

Second, there are teachers who feel convinced that real

learning only takes place through direct teaching of subject matter; such teaching strategies are concrete and measurable and give a teacher a sense of power and security.

Finally, there are the social pressures toward hurrying children to which Elkind (1981) and others (Miller, 1981; Packard, 1983) have been recently alerting us. Parents and teachers seem driven by these pressures to focus on cognitive development and achievements without recognizing the intertwining of the affective with the cognitive which can retard or facilitate development.

It is interesting that the phenomenon of the non-playing child is occurring when the literature on play has mushroomed in the past decade. This literature demonstrates that there are a large number of cognitive, social, and emotional payoffs for the playing child (see Fein, 1981 for an excellent and comprehensive review). Another body of knowledge deals with the importance of the first 3 years of life for the establishment of a firm sense of self (e.g., Erikson, 1950; Greenspan & Greenspan, 1985; Kaplan, 1978; Mahler et al., 1975; Piaget & Inhelder, 1969; Sander, 1975). In this paper I will attempt:

1. To link the symbol systems of play and language to the development of the sense of self with the recognition that these symbol systems both mirror and enhance the evolution of the self;
2. To highlight the value of playful, affectively charged interchanges between caregivers and children; and
3. To propose an intervention model for caregivers when children seem developmentally delayed in terms of language and play. This model is built on playful interactions which parallel what the "good enough" mother (Winnicott, 1965) does to enhance the optimal self-development of her child.

PLAY AND THE DEVELOPING SENSE OF SELF

By referring to the first 3 years of life as the time for "psychological birth of the human infant" Mahler et al. (1975) bring into focus the importance of these years for the development of a solid sense of self. Sander (1975), using an interaction approach, outlines seven adaptational issues in the first 3 years of life which parallel to a certain extent the subphases of separation-individuation as explicated by Mahler. (See Foley in this issue for a succinct condensation of the Mahler's separation-individuation process with some modifications.) This section will focus on the play indicators that both mirror and enhance the progress the child makes toward self-definition during the first 3 years of life. Dramatic play is defined as "a unifying force by which the child's social and physical experiences with the external world are integrated with internal mental and emotional processes to produce novel transformations which are then projected outward in symbolic form" (Curry, 1972, pp. 124–25). The role parents play in this unifying process through emotionally laden interchanges will be highlighted.

Birth to Three Months

The earliest affective interchanges between parent and child involve caregiving, language and play. In this early period, which Mahler et al. (1975) label *relative autism,* Sander (1975) calls *initial regulation,* and Foley (1986) designates *naive synchrony,* infants and their families are learning to live together. The baby sends out beginning signals which parents learn to read and to respond to through predictable ministrations usually accompanied by playful words, sounds and gestures. In essence, the stage is being set and the cast is being assembled for the child's play and affective life. Brazelton and Als (1979, p. 366) trace a developmental beginning play sequence for this period:

1. Physiological motor orientation and state regulation during which the baby alternately shuts out and reaches for stimuli;
2. Orientation in which the child begins to prolong attention states;
3. Play dialogue;
4. Beginning of object play.

Parents facilitate this development by evoking their babies' beginning awareness of what comes from inside themselves and what comes from the outside through predictable caregiving and through play episodes of vocalizing, echoing their children's vocalizations and responding to their babies' cues by either decreasing or increasing stimulation. Brazelton and Als (1979) speak of the value of parents pressing the limits of child's capacity to take in during these play times, and then permitting the child to withdraw to recover homeostasis. They stress that the real test of attachement is demonstrated by these play sequences that culminate near the end of the 3rd or 4th month as play with toy objects begins.

Four to Nine Months

Mahler et al. (1975) label this period as the *differentiation* subphase. Children begin to differentiate themselves and to particularize the meaningful people in their lives. There is a new look of alertness on their faces as they take in every aspect of the widening world. As they achieve eye/hand/mouth coordination, a period of intense exploration begins which includes exploring their own body parts and functions along with the manual, tactile, and visual explorations of mother's face and body as well as of toys and space. Mother-infant reciprocal play emerges during caregiving functions and continues to involve much touching and vocalizing with parents mirroring and extending the child's activities.

Parents facilitate the burgeoning individuality of their children at this time in the age-old games of babyhood. Naming and touching body parts "Where's baby's nose?", nursery rhymes, such as "This little piggy", and games of peek-a-boo help parents tell their children in symbolic form "this is me and this is you." Catch-me games begin as the child becomes more mobile with the parent as the initiator and catcher ("I'm gonna get you") and the baby as catchee. Games such as tossing toys to the floor also make their appearance; parents learn to be patient with the children's seemingly endless fascination with this beginning separation game. The introduction of objects with a variety of sensory-modalities aid in the more impersonal differentiation tasks that are a part of this exciting period. Most parents are comfortable with their children's exploration of their (the parents) bodies (touching and pulling at hair, ears, eyes and noses). They also continually emotionally invest their children's bodies through vestibular experiences of lifting, swinging, pulling and jumping games. The child's exploratory urgency is supported and highlighted by parents who offer a running commentary through what Schachter et al. (1976) call "alter ego talk" (p. 221); the naming, labeling, interpreting, and commenting that parents do with their babies. This "alter ego talk" calls the child's attention to himself/herself as the actor and helps integrate the actor and his/her acts through words.

Nine to Eighteen Months

In the *practicing* period (Mahler et al., 1975), infants begin to show more independence and directed exploration as their locomotive functions develop at a rapid rate. There is an air of purposefulness about their play as they creep around touching, tasting, and feeling or as they experience periods of "alert inactivity," visually scanning their environment. Harvard studies have shown that the extended periods of "focussed staring" are characteristic of 2-year-olds rated high in competency (Gould, 1972). The beginnings of a sense of potency arise with the child's taking great pleasure in being the initiator and doer in play. With an intense investment in locomotive play, the primary mood is that of elation (Mahler et al., 1975) or what Greenacre (1957) describes as "a love affair with the world." Mahler et al. (1975) also note the "low-keyed" behavior of the practicing child which is induced by parents' unavailability, either physical or emotional. Taunting parents into games of run and chase demonstrate children's thrust toward independence, but also the inexorable need to be reassured that their parents will come after them.

In addition to their involvement in physical play and exploration, the infants are creating and comprehending a wide variety of symbols, with the outstanding example being language. Their receptive language and rudimentary imitative play show the dawning capacity to deal with abstractions (i.e., a word can stand for an object, feeling, event, person, place, or activity). Prior to the time children use these symbols in expressive language, they use playful gestures which, again, are demonstrative of the ability to interact symbolically with the widening world, provided the ability has been reinforced by loving caregivers who continue to integrate the child's playful activities with language.

The parents' play contributions during the practicing period remain crucial. In addition to the multifaceted roles of safe base, limit-setter, introducer of new experience, mediator, and role model, parents intensify their interpretive function. They quite intuitively reinforce their children's sense of potency by reporting and reflecting the children's activities and feelings: "You're playing with the ball"; "You'd like to try to climb the stairs"; "You're tired. You've had a busy day." Such natural comments tell the children that their activities are worthwhile, that they themselves are of great value to their caregivers, and that their feeling states are perceived, understood, acted on, and respected.

Eighteen to Twenty-Four Months

Mahler et al. (1975) delinate the *rapprochement* period which has deepened our understanding of this developmental crossroad which Erikson (1950) earlier alerted us to as the crisis between *autonomy* and *self-doubt.* Emotionally, the push toward independence and the seductive pull back to dependence create an ambitendency that is reflected in all facets of the child's behavior, including play (Mahler et al., 1975). The two major symbolic systems of language and play flower at this time and, in fact, confront children with the cognitive awareness of separateness.

Thus, the second year of life is a nodal one for all developing children. Witness the developmental foundation for expressive and receptive language that Helen Keller established prior to her illness at 17 months on which she could later build. Once her teacher helped her rediscover the usefulness of language she was able to use it depthfully and creatively throughout her life (Fraiberg, 1977). Both Mahler et al. (1975) and Piaget (1959) point out that there is a shift from primarily sensorimotor play to beginning symbolic play with language as a second symbol system. As receptive and expressive language capacities grow, children can indicate needs, wishes, and feelings symbolically rather than by acting them out directly. Further differentiation of self from others is made possible by language. A child seems to realize: I create the words, I see the other people, objects, and things have labels and I can use these labels in a common symbolic system that makes me a part of the world around me, at the same time as I am finding that I exist separately in that world. The era of symbolic play begins to emerge when people are perceived more clearly and, therefore, are classified for the playing youngsters as they try out what they do through representational play acts. A tattered scarf draped over one's head can symbolize mother, children can now tolerate mother's absence by imitating her activities or appearance. A briefcase can represent Daddy or Mother and when lugged about endows children with some of the attributes of power seen all around in those grownups essential for the child's existence. Once again, as in the development of speech, such play acts indicate that children are beginning to see other people as separate from themselves just as they, with their growing capacity to symbolize, are becoming autonomous beings. Curiosity and exploration run as rampant as do young toddlers as they reach out to the environment in playful encounters.

Parents need to understand the dynamics of the behavior of their ambivalent youngsters, so they can respond empathically rather than assume their youngsters may be inherently bad ("He's just like Uncle Charlie") or out to get them ("She *knows* I can't stand temper tantrums"). They help by channeling their children's intense emotionality and curiosity into purposeful play and by continuing to reflect and comment on the children's activities which teach them about their world and how they fit (or sometimes don't fit) into it. They absorb children's sometimes overwhelming affect ("I know you are angry, but I can't let you hurt the baby or me. Let's build up your block tower again and you can knock that down"), offer play alternatives to the binds children get themselves into ("Let's put your teddy to bed, and then you can lie down and help him go to sleep"), and help children master the intensity of a situation by casting it in a playful mold ("You can give the dolly a shot, like Dr. S. gave one to you today"). They supply opportunities for symbolization for their children's developmental conflicts and interest around separation and individuation: games of disappearance and reappearance, toys that elicit representative play, tasks of sorting and discrimination, or emptying and filling play. They deepen their roles as audience to their playing children who desperately need the mirroring approval of parents at a time when they are torn by powerful emotions in themselves which may feel unacceptable.

Schachter and her colleagues (Schachter et al., 1976; Schachter, 1979), in studying the verbal interactions between children both with caregivers in day care classes and with parents in their homes, have delineated the predominantly alter-ego speech of caregivers toward toddlers and the later ego-supportive and ego-socializing speech with 3-and 4-year-olds. In evaluating the responsive and spontaneous speech acts of educated mothers (both black and white) and disadvantaged mothers (black) Schachter (1979) concludes,

> Our results indicate that the educated mothers take the affective development of their toddlers into account. They support their toddlers' emerging autonomy, helping them attain their own goals; validating their own observations and experiences; boosting their nascent egos; minimizing prohibitions and providing justifications or substitutes when restrictions are necessary; and teaching when the child's interest is engaged. . . . The responsive communication style of our educated mothers seems to consist of a set of strategies that support the burgeoning selfhood of the toddler. (p. 93)

Two to Three Year Olds

To refer to this age span as one of the consolidation of beginning play and language skills and of the sense of self is to minimize the tremendous richness of this period. In sum, Mahler et al. (1975) elaborate on what occurs during the late rapprochement period leading to libidinal object constancy. This means the youngster can tolerate separation because of an internal image of the parents. To recognize that one can be good and bad and still be the same person is a hallmark of self-constancy; to realize that the people one loves and depends upon can also be good and bad at the same time leads to a sense of *their* constancy. In Mahler's et al. (1975) terms, there is an experiential sense of their constancy regardless of how one feels about them or regardless of their physical presence or absence. As children attain this sense of self-and-other libidinal object constancy, their energies become more fully available for symbolizing experiences through language and through play.

While the sensorimotor, exploratory play continues, along with the ego activities of empty and filling, building and knocking down, appearance and disappearance, pushing and pulling (Freud, 1965), fantasy role and pretend play deepens. If all has gone well between parent and child, the child can play out both nurturing and aggressive roles (Gould, 1972) with greater emphasis on the nurturant-provider. Dyadic play of mother/baby, doctor/patient, adult/baby animals, big/little sister or brother, emerges with *some* reciprocal alternation. Generally, aggression themes are less well developed because most 2-year-olds attempting these themes become so flooded with affect that they cannot use their cognitive capacities for distancing and symbolizing.

Parents continue their alter ego functions and move into an ego-enhancing mode as well (Schachter et al., 1976). The richly unfolding play and language repertoires of the child call for a wider range of responses from caregivers. The enlarging capacity for pretend play is facilitated by adults who model the role of a playful person, who engage in pretend play with zest, and who bestow their approval on the playing child ("You're playing house so well today"). By supplying props, developmentally appropriate peers, and well-timed commentaries and suggestions, adults let the child know that playful pretence is an activity that has meaning and value.

THE VALUE OF DRAMATIC PLAY

Most writers are in agreement that pretend or dramatic play is at its height during the preschool years (Fein, 1981; Piaget, 1962 Smilansky, 1968). For the normally developing child, by age 3 depthful dramatic play has begun to serve an integrative function in the symbolic process. In rudimentary dramatic play, children depict representationally that which they have observed or experienced and in the process symbolize both external and internal reality (Curry, 1972). To be able to produce a play action that stands for or replicates a real emotion (pretending to be angry) or event (pretending that it's bedtime by covering oneself or a teddy bear) is a further step in abstraction. Children symbolize through a variety of symbolic channels: art, language, block-building, dramatic play.

This natural mode of self-expression involves a variety of complex learning strategies. To develop and maintain a depthful dramatic play episode, one must be able to convey to one's fellow players the salient aspects of the role being portrayed. This involves having comprehended the essence of the person or animal one is playing, not only by imitating the physical appearance, stance and activities of the model, but also by portraying its feelings and reactions. Furthermore, if the playing child, is to have satisfying, continuing sociodramatic play (Smilansky, 1968), he must have some understanding of the role being portrayed by the other child or children who are contributing to the drama. This requires memory, empathy, and the capacity to see something from another's point of view as well as the ability to concentrate, to stay in role, and to maintain the stance of pretending to be another person while still being one's self. All these skills imply the attainment of at least some reversibility and conservation in Piaget's sense as well as a sense of self. Gould (1972) has given us an excellent framework for examining the intertwining of affect and cognition expressed in symbolic play. Parents aid in the integration of affect and cognition by commenting and labeling their child's ongoing activities and feeling states, thus enhancing the child's sense of being an active, effective self.

MODEL OF PLAY INTERVENTION

To return to my question, where have all the players gone, I believe they are very much with us, but may be stifled by social, emotional, and environmental factors. Three of the environmental factors may well be the educational goals, attitudes and strategies of both parents and teachers. In returning to the clinical impressions described at the beginning of this paper, (the lack of play and language skills of some disadvantaged preschoolers and the lack of play and language interchanges between poor young mothers and their babies), one finds support in the literature from observations and research of others. For example, Schachter (1979) in her summary of the comparison of language interchanges between educated black and white mothers and their children and poor black mothers and their children found:

> Indeed, in many respects, the disadvantaged mother resembles the caregivers in didactic programs . . . she initiates most of her daily verbal interactions with the child; her speech is dominated by control talk and teaching talk; she makes frequent use of negative commands; she emphasizes the teaching of letters and numbers; and she often uses the technique of exact self-repetition. Like these teachers she generally talks *to* the child rather than responsively *with* the child. (p. 154)

In the Oxford study of preschool teaching conducted by Bruner and reported on in a series of exciting books (Bruner, 1980; Sylva, Roy and Painter, 1980; Wood, McMahon & Cranstoun, 1980), the teaching styles of teachers were delineated through their own recordings of their everyday encounters with children. In their observational studies of teacher-pupil interactions, when teachers were confronted with their everyday interactions with children, they were horrified.

> Indeed the tendency to ignore children, talk over and then generally dominate the proceedings, was the single most striking feature of the recordings that our 24 practitioners responded to when they read their transcripts. Many were appalled and surprised by the blinkering effect that their own questions had on their attention to what children were saying. (Wood et al., 1980, p. 85)

These studies supply us with both antecedent and concurrent factors that influence the depth and breadth of play development. So, what can we do as child caring professionals? A developmental framework gives us guidelines to diagnose where a child might be on the developmental play continuum and to design interventions appropriate for that developmental level. An interventive program is proposed which emphasizes the role of the caregiver, although the author recognizes that play can be equally facilitated by the environment and other children (Curry & Arnaud, 1984). Theoretical background to this proposed interventive program comes from the separation-individuation studies of Mahler and her colleagues (1975), from the interactional language studies and parent training program of Schachter and her colleagues (Schachter et al., 1976; Schachter, 1979), from a training program in modeling language and play for parents of retarded children (Seitz & Hoekenga, 1974), from Smilansky's model for play interaction (1968), and from psychotherapy literature (Axline, 1947; Greenson, 1967; Brady and Friedrich, 1982). All of these authors stress the importance of the adult's commenting on and reflecting the child's (or patient's) activities. The adult serves as an alter ego and an ego enhancer (Schachter et al., 1976) by highlighting the value of and extending the child's productions. Implementing this approach with disadvantged preschoolers in the classroom and in therapeutic play sessions shows promise both for developing play and language skills and for bolstering the child's burgeoning sense of self.

Organizing the Environment

For example, for children who appear completely disorganized and chaotic, even in the basic tasks of living such as eating and sleeping, one may need to begin with organizing their world for them much as a mother does for a baby in the first 3 months of age, the normal period of *initial regulation* (Sander, 1975). Creating a predictable environment for children includes keeping materials in predictable spots, having routines which seldom vary, and using one's body as a safe home base, and may assist a severely regressed child in developing the basic regularity that most very young infants achieve as a matter of course.

Aiding in Differentiation

If children demonstrate that they have little, if any, sense of who they are in relation to the rest of the world, one can speculate that the period of differentiation presented difficulties. Such children do not seem to recognize themselves in a mirror, have difficulty with the pronouns "I" or "me", and seem incapable of concentrated attention. One may need to play with such a child much as a mother would a 4- to 6 month-old baby: encourage mutual body play; touch and name the child's body parts; and permit the child to explore the caregiver's own face, hair, jewelry and clothing. Games of peek-a-boo are useful, as is using the mirror in which the child sees two people (her/himself and the teacher) with the end goal being to differentiate each person, "This is you and this is me."

Narrating the Child's Activities

If the child seems stuck in the motor practicing period with such behavior as "run and chase" (Speers, 1974), it may be necessary for the caregiver to serve as an organizer much as the mother does during the practicing period of 9 to 15 months. Thus, the nonplaying child in a preschool may benefit from having the caregiver narrate the child's activities in a fashion similar to mother. For example, the teacher might sit with the child in the doll corner and make a running commentary on the child's activities. "You are putting the dishes on the stove. You are giving the baby a bite of the cookie. Now you are taking the baby for a ride in the stroller." This commentary helps the child organize and process cognitively what is going on. At the same time the caregiver can narrate for the child what the other playing children are doing, both to provide integration of what the child is seeing and hearing and to indicate her approval of play in general. "Johnny and Mark are playing doctor. Johnny is using the stethoscope. It makes Mark laugh—maybe it tickles."

Joining in the Play

Once children begin to supply their own narration of their ongoing activities (as most average 3-year-olds do spontaneously), the caregiver can take on a role in the play. Smilansky's (1968) work has been pioneering in this area. She suggests that the teacher try intervening either outside the play (by describing what is going on and suggesting a role for that child) or by joining in the play ("Pretend I'm grandma and I came to visit. This could be our house"). It is important to keep the pretend activities within the child's range of play experience (e.g., feeding, bedtime, trips to the store or doctor) and watch closely for when the child begins to show initiative. With most children, the adult need not stay in the play forever; once the child gets energized, and can play independently the caregiver can sit nearby and comment on the child's actions and reflect the feelings he may be experiencing.

Utilizing Other Children

Once the child has the rudiments of pretend play, it is useful to get other children involved with him. "You made me such good cookies. Let's see if Megan would like some for her house," or "Your He-Man castle is great. I'll bet Tammy would like to be Tela." Once two or more children become involved with each other, they will not be distracted by other competing activities if adults continue to call them by role names and provide occasional comments on their actions (Curry and Arnaud, 1984).

Intervening at Cognitive and Emotional Levels

Even good players experience breakdowns in their play or fail to get a play episode off the ground. When this happens in the preschool setting, they may not have an adult who takes their play seriously, or who may not want to invest herself in the play situation. In line with the earlier suggestions for non-playing children, the teacher's attitude toward play (i.e., that it is a valuable and necessary curricular tool) and her teaching style (Schachter's alter ego and ego-supportive speech styles, 1979) will advance and deepen dramatic play bouts.

When disruptions occur, they usually are the result of either emotional or cognitive interferences (Tittnich, 1984). Here the child's affective development comes into sharp focus. The inability to distinguish between real and make-believe and the inability to distance and display one's feeling in symbolic role play often occur in children with a shaky sense of self (Gould, 1972). Often their role play gets disrupted when anxiety becomes overwhelming. When the teacher perceives that there are emotional interferences, she can intervene through supplying ego supportive clarifications and suggestions as exemplified here:

1. Yes, He-Man does attack Skeletor sometimes, but he also has to have a place to live. Do you think you could make a castle out of these blocks?
2. You started building a fine railroad and Billy knocked your station over. He and I will help you get it built again so your passengers will have a place to wait. Where have you decided to take your train?
3. Johnny's pretending to be a tiger, but his growling scared you. Maybe you could be the zookeeper and make a cage for him.

If the teacher perceives that the interference comes from cognitive misunderstandings or gaps, she can gear her facilitating comments to address them. Examples of teacher's responses to cognitive interferences are:

1. You seem to be having trouble getting started playing Burger Chef. You can decide who will be the cook, who will be the customer, and who is going to take the order. Your building could have a drive-through window here.
2. I hear your baby crying, Mother. Do you think she needs to see the doctor? Jimmy is playing doctor over there and he needs some patients.
3. You were wanting to play store yesterday and we ran out of time. I've brought in some boxes and toy fruits and vegetables and the new cash register. This area could be your store and Melissa and Sally still need to buy food for their party.

With this basic developmental approach caregivers can participate and cooperate in order to move the child forward. The strategies that I have described certainly involve activities which are commonly engaged in by parents during the very early developmental stages. If children without these earlier interpersonal experiences with parents continue to call out comparable interactive styles from their teachers, as Wood et al. (1980) point out, they will continue to fall behind in the play and language skills which are necessary "for successful integration into the school situations or full cooperation in the 'school game' " (Smilansky, 1968, p. 42).

On the whole, caregivers may be more accustomed to and more comfortable with educational techniques which are geared to the child's cognitive capacities. Yet children thrive on the loving investments made by adults as they move through the stages leading to a solid sense of self. Play, in addition to being highly pleasurable and a natural mode for young children, integrates cognitive and affective aspects of development. Caring adults, as catalysts in the integrative process, supply the opportunities and encouragement to play, and the language and other nutriments necessary to facilitate the synthetic functions of play.

SUMMARY

In this paper, I have described the developmental framework within which the child separates and individuates. Further, I have attempted to trace the progress the child makes toward abstract thinking and the functions of language and dramatic play in the symbolic process. These developmental landmarks can become diagnostic tools when we are dealing with children who show developmental lags in terms of play, language and/or self development. Interventive strategies modeled on parents' roles as organizers and facilitators have been suggested with a focus on the use of language and affectively-tinged playful exchanges to consolidate self-development.

REFERENCES

Axline, V. (1947). *Play therapy*. Boston: Houghton Mifflin.

Baldwin, A. & Baldwin, C. (1973). The study of mother-child interaction. *American Scientist, 61,* 714–721.

Bee, H.L., Van Egeren, L.F., Streissguth, A.P., Nyman, B.A., & Leckie, M.S. (1969). Social class differences in maternal teaching strategies and speech patterns. *Developmental Psychology, 1,* 726–734.

Bjorkland, G. (1978). *Planning for play: A developmental approach.* Columbus, OH: Charles Merrill.

Brady, C.A. & Friedrich, W.N. (1982). Levels of intervention: A model for training in play therapy. *Journal of Clinical Child Psychology,* 11:1, 39–43.

Brazelton, T.B. & Als, H. (1979). Four early stages in the development of mother-infant interaction. In *Psychoanalytic study of the child, 34,* 349–370.

Bruner, J. (1980). *Under five in Britain.* Ypsilanti: High Scope.

Curry, N.E. (1972). *Current issues in play: Theoretical and practical considerations for its use as a curricular tool in the preschool.* Unpublished doctoral dissertation.

Curry, N.E. & Arnaud, S.H. (1984). Play in developmental preschool settings. In T.D. Yawkey, & A.D. Pellegrini (Eds.), *Child's play* (pp. 273–290). Hillsdale, NJ: Lawrence Erlbaum.

Elkind, D. (1981). *The hurried child.* Reading, Mass: Addison-Wesley.

Erikson, E.H. (1950). *Childhood & society.* New York: Norton.

Fein, G. (1981). Pretend play in childhood: An integrative review. *Child Development, 52,* 1095–1118.

Foley, G. (1986). Emotional development of handicapped children. *Journal of Children in Contemporary Society, 17*(4).

Fraiberg, S. (1977). *Insight from the blind: Developmental studies of blind children.* New York: Basic Books.

Freud, A. (1965). *Normality and pathology in childhood.* New York: International Universities Press.

Gould, R. (1972). *Child studies through fantasy.* New York: Quadrangle Books.

Greenacre, P. (1957). The childhood of the artist: Libidinal phase development and giftedness. *The Psychoanalytic Study of the Child, 12,* 27–72.

Greenspan, S. & Greenspan, N.T. (1985). *First feelings.* New York: Viking Penguin.

Greenson, R.R. (1967). *The technique and practice of psychoanalysis.* New York: International Universities Press.

Hess, R. & Shipman, V.C. (1965). Early experience on the socialization of cognitive modes in children. *Child Development, 34,* 869–886.

Kaplan, L.J. (1978). *Oneness & separateness: From infant to individual.* New York: Simon & Shuster.

Mahler, M., Pine, F. & Bergman, A. (1975) *The psychological birth of the human infant.* New York: Basic Books.

Miller, A. (1981). *Prisoners of childhood.* New York: Basic Books.

Packard, V. (1983). *Our endangered children.* Boston: Little, Brown.

Piaget, J. (1959). *The language and thought of the child* (3rd. ed.) New York: Humanities Press.

Piaget, J. (1962). *Play, dreams and imitation in childhood.* New York: Norton. (original work published 1951).

Piaget, J. & Inhelder, B. (1969). *The psychology of the child.* New York: Basic Books.

Sander, L. (1975). Infant and caretaking environment. In J. Anthony (Ed). *Explorations in child psychiatry* (pp. 129–164). New York: Plenum.

Schachter, F.F. (1979). *Everyday mother talk to toddlers: Early intervention.* New York: Academic Press.

Schachter, F.F., Fosha, D., Stemp, S., Brotman, N., & Ganger, S. (1976). Everyday caretaker talk to toddlers vs. three and fours. *Journal of Child Language, 3,* 221–245.

Seitz, S. & Hoekenga, R. (1974). Modeling as a training tool for retarded children and their parents. *Mental Retardation, 12,* 28–31.

Smilansky, S. (1968). *The effects of sociodramatic play on disadvantaged preschool children.* New York: John Wiley.

Snow C.E., Arlman-Rupp, A., Hassing, Y., Jobse, J., Joosten, J., & Vorster, J. (1976). Mothers' speech in three social classes. *Journal Psycholinguistic Research, 5,* 1–19.

Speers, R.W. (1974). Variations in separation-individuation and implications for play ability and learning. In D. Bergsma, R.T. Gross, C.F. Settlage, A.J. Solnit, and D. Dwyer (Eds.) *The infant at risk* (pp. 77–100). New York: Intercontinental Medical Book Corp.

Spitz, R.A. (1965). *The first year of life.* New York: International Universities Press.
Sylva, K., Roy, C., & Painter, M. (1980). *Child watching at play group and nursery school.* Ypsilanti: High Scope.
Tittnich, E.T. (1984). Personal communication.
Winnicott, D.W. (1965). *The maturation processes and the facilitating environment.* London: Hogarth.
Wood, D., McMahon, L., & Cranstoun, Y. (1980). *Working with under fives.* Ypsilanti: High Scope.

Helping Children in Times of Trouble and Crisis

Victoria Jean Dimidjian, PhD

ABSTRACT. This paper highlights the impact of personal and social crisis in the lives of young children and distinguishes categories of potential stress in today's world. Examination of various roles and actions of helping adults in assisting children to adaptively confront personal and social crisis provides illustration of how parents, teachers, and other helping adults can affirm innate resiliency while simultaneously strengthening understanding.

INTRODUCTION

"Crisis?" echoed the new nursery school teacher as the others sitting around the table watched her begin to respond to the question.

> That word . . . I remember when we first studied Erikson's stages and psychosocial crises. At first, the idea of "crisis" was so abstract. Then I began to see the pushes and pulls in other's lives. Mine too. . . . But this year, my first time teaching, like helping live wire Matthew get ready for the surgery and then getting reestablished in the class afterwards . . . or seeing the effects of two different families pulling apart, the tears and troubles that came up so often in class during those months . . . and then this spring when our children couldn't get into the church entrance for nursery school because the unemployed steelworkers were picketing! I *never* imagined I'd be asked to help children and families with that!

Victoria Jean Dimidjian is Associate Professor, Director of Early Childhood Education and Chair of Women's Studies Department at Carlow College, 3333 Fifth Avenue, Pittsburgh, PA 15213. Reprints may be obtained from the author.

She looked around the table at her nodding friends, graduates, and fellow first-year teachers. One, a young man working as a day care supervisor, talked of his struggles encountering his first case of child abuse. Then he described examples of cooperative work with families such as helping a non-English speaking child start day care successfully and assisting a now drug-free mother begin to encourage her child's skills at home as teachers did in the center. "Crisis?" he echoed too. "The solutions on TV are so pat, that's phony, for sure, but the crises there aren't fake. I already feel old saying this, but kids growing up in times like these, that's almost a crisis in itself! Makes me really think again about whether I want to start a family, I tell you . . . ," And the conversation moved to discussion of personal critical decisions facing this group of young professionals.

Whether as parent, teacher, therapist, involved adult, or as some patchwork patterning of several of these roles, adults looking protectively at today's young note the predominant number who encounter crises, often on a too-regular and recurrent basis, throughout their formative years. *Crisis:* a period of decisive change, a time of acute difficulty and potential danger producing marked change in the post-crisis period. As Erikson (1950, 1968) has described, human development occurs in a series of developmental thrusts toward resolution of psychosocial polarities. Even in the most nurturing, stable, and stimulating home or community environments, the growing child pulsates with expressions of energetic stress as he or she stretches toward ever-fuller growth.

However, the contemporary culture in local communities and across the globe rarely offers growth conditions consistently characterized as nurturing, stable and stimulating. Instead, individual adults and their collective social structures appear too often to be connected by sheerest gossamer threads. Social fabrics and individual lives are all too easily rent by the stress of social change, political dissension, economic stress or interpersonal conflict between social subgroups.

This paper begins by distinguishing the categories of stress and possible crisis which can impact on growing lives in today's world. Utilizing Bronfenbrenner's (1979) ecological conception of the interacting spheres of influence in children's lives, contrasts are presented from crisis in personal, communal and societal domains, all of which impact stressfully on the young. Then examination of the various roles and actions of helping adults ensues, illustrating appropriate methods of assisting the child in continuing to grow and adaptively confront, perhaps even engage in attempts to repair, the environmental fabric of the social world while solidifying affective stability.

CONCEPTUALIZING CRISIS IN CHILDREN'S LIVES

Daily encounters with children bring every adult into awareness of the critical changes posed so early and so strongly to those just beginning to form coherent understanding of the world around them. For example, a 4-year-old eating dinner with her parents says, "Sandy was crying at school today. Her daddy's in the hospital. She said he got mugged last night. What's mugged?" Or an 8-year-old returning to school on Monday tells his teacher about Saturday afternoon at the playground, about "the big fight" between a gang of older boys and the police, the knife one boy pulled, the shouting and hitting that, he says, "went on and on." Or a 12-year-old leaves on a commercial break to run upstairs and get her old "blankie," then returns to the TV with the rest of the family circled there. But now she sits enclosed in the blanket, within the comfort of her parent's arm as they watch "The Day After." Afterwards they talk, but that night she is unable to sleep until much of the night has disappeared. Thus children show that they register the impact of personal, social, even global crisis in their questions, discussions, creative expressions, and often through dreams and fantasies.

In understanding and helping children cope, it is important for the adult to distinguish the parameters of crisis which have or are currently having an impact on the child. Utilizing Bronfenbrenner's (1979) ecological framework for interacting spheres of influence on children's lives, Table I presents this author's conceptual framework for distinguishing the realms of crisis growing children may encounter. From the contrasting examples presented in Table I, it is clear that in addition to the ecological setting which defines the parameters of the critical stress, the second differentiating factor is timeframe. Sudden

Table 1: Domains of Crisis Impacting on Children's Lives

Sphere	Timeframe	Examples
Microsystem (self/familial world)	Sudden, immediate duration	Severe personal injury Unexpected death of family member Sudden severing of family bonds or marked change in family structure
	Progressive, shorter duration	Onset and treatment of a potentially disabling health condition Divorce
	Progressive, longer duration	Expectation and birth of new sibling Surgery for treatment of chronic health condition Remarriage of a parent and/or reformation of family structure
Mesosystem (Child/family embedded in larger community bonds)	Sudden, immediate duration	Unexpected death of community leader (principal, minister/rabbi, mayor Catastrophic natural disaster, e.g., flood, fire, tornado Unemployment of family supporter(s) Group or mob violence
	Progressive, shorter duration	Move to new home, neighborhood, or school Mainstreaming of disabled child previously placed in special setting
	Progressive, longer duration	Forced merging of school districts or human service institutions Ongoing social stress with intermittent strife between groups in community
Macrosystem (Child/family/community within national and global bonds)	Sudden, immediate duration	Assassination of political or social leader Large-scale natural disaster (e.g., earthquake or flood) Large-scale humanmade disaster (e.g., Hiroshima, Nagasaki, The Holocaust)
	Progressive, shorter duration	Economic turndown or depression Economic transition from agricultural base to industrial base to technological base Health epidemic or threatened epidemic
	Progressive, longer duration	Threat of nuclear annihilation Extended wars between nation states or large social groups within the nations continents Large-scale natural disaster (e.g., drought and famine in Subsahara or Cambodia)

change such as the loss of a parent in an automobile accident or the unexpected onset of a stressful condition such as a flood or tornado in an area where such occurrences have never happened causes greater demands on the resiliency and adaptability of either the individual or the social system than do critical stresses which have developed progressively and allowed a preparatory period for initiation of coping behaviors.

Whatever the source(s) precipitating the crisis and the particular dynamic situation, the dangerous potential remains similar for all classes of stress: that adaptive coping with the challenge will not be possible and that the child's intellectual and/or socioemotional growth will be inhibited, even stunted. Like Freud's characterization of the healthy adult as one who can work and love effectively, so the healthy child may be characterized as one who is able to develop progressively and simultaneously thinking, feeling and acting skills and to manifest these skills in play and goal-directed activities in home, school or community. Traumatic and poorly resolved crisis can interfere or block such development as decades of case histories of children in treatment since 1900 aptly illustrate.

Crisis in Microsystem of Self/Familial World

Works of Furman (1974, 1978), for example, in the area of childhood bereavement provide a thorough picture of the mourning process and the resolution of the loss of a parent that is undertaken by children in varying developmental stages. *A Child's Parent Dies* (1974) contrasts George and Mark, both boys who lost their parents by suicide during the preschool period. In George's family the loss was so sudden, traumatic, and painful that his mourning process could not be completed. Mark's family too was deeply shaken by the traumatic loss through self-destruction. In this case, however, the community and therapeutic supports made individual and family system mourning possible. Although not completed for some years after the initial loss, Mark was finally able to complete the mourning process and resolve the trauma, without defensively forgetting it or anxiously replaying it or searching for the lost parent.

Crisis in Mesosystem and Macrosystem Domains

Kliman et al. (1965) have also studied effects of parental loss, but additionally they have examined immediate and longer-term responses to loss of a national leader through assassination. In their work with children of varying age levels following John Kennedy's death, children's coping capacities are clearly contrasted depending on previous life experience, developmental status and responses of the adult environment.

In a later work, Kliman (1968) points to a paradigm of the helping environment in coping with loss of national leader stating:

> In this particular national psychological emergency and in the management of the children within it are seen the same major principles which usually apply in cases of family tragedy. Generally, the sooner a child knows, the better he absorbs the news; the more participation in adult reaction, the better; the more opportunity to react with adult and peer support, the better; the more organized and supportive the adult-structured environment, the better. (p. 136)

Yet it is only in the late 20th Century that conditions of personal, community, and global life has become so technologically interconnected that the possibility now exists for multiple levels of trauma to occur or recur. Terr's (1979) study of the children of Chowchilla evidences the severely stressed, sometimes traumatized, reactions of 23 California children who were kidnapped and buried in 1976. Her work illustrates how the resiliency of all children was shaken, particularly so with children whose attempts to meet stress and crisis were incomplete and unsupported by adults. During this period the author witnessed two children in day care centers repetitively playing "kidnapping," seeming to echo, the media attention and parental concern that such an incident evoked. Similarly, this author currently has noted expression as "kidnapping" fears in children as national attention has been increasingly highlighting the disappearance of a small although important number of young children.

This connection between cultural levels and their impact on a child facing crisis was especially exemplified in this author's work with a 4.6-year-old boy attending a day care center in his congested, poverty-packed, factory-bound community. He had lived with his single mother and disabled grandparents all his life. His family system provided some sense of security but was often near the edge of survival due to mother's insecure employment status. Both grandparents were deeply involved in caring for the child since birth. At age 4 this boy witnessed his grandfather being stricken by heart failure and removed by ambulance to the local hospital where he died. This boy literally vibrated with tension as sirens sounded outside his day care classroom, and he repetitively played "ambulance" and "emergency" episodes in the dramatic play corner with increasing self-involved roles, often ignoring initiatives of teachers or other children. At home, he oriented TV-watching around "emergency" programs and even at age 4 zeroed in on medical trauma in local news. For the first several weeks in treatment, his play was tentative, disjointed, and his words touched on many topics except that of loss. Not until facing a short break in sessions did he turn to me in tears, saying, "*Why* do you always have to say goodbyes? Why does everybody always go goodbyes?" After the first direct expression in these words of his "big boy questions and little boy panicky feelings," we were then able to begin work on the loss he had so traumatically suffered and continued to suffer as he reinvoked it in the "emergencies" which periodically invaded his life.

Helpless, fixated re-echoing of trauma is also illustrated in an example provided by McQuade (1985) whose consultation was requested by a preschool mainstreaming a physically handicapped girl.[1] Teachers there were concerned about overtures she made after initial adjustment to her new classroom. During her first on-site observation, the consultant noticed the child's rigid body posture as she stood unmoving beside the water table, her expression frozen and fingers clenched on the edge. On close examination of the water table, the consultant saw a dismembered doll floating among the other toys. The consultant discussed this with the head teacher, stressing the need for intact, well-functioning materials for this child particularly and the necessity of adult support when unforeseen stress situations occurred. With caring adult support, the child was later able to repair "broken things" and to develop increasingly adaptive and active behaviors. However, her locked-in-fear reactions to starving children shown on the TV news or to disfigured monsters in films may go unnoticed by adults who fail to engage in empathic reflection about "why" her facial muscles tense or her body goes rigid in anxiety-inducing situations.

The adult's goal in helping children to cope with crisis, then, is to assist the child in developing adaptive behaviors founded on understanding, ultimately resulting in the child's responsible, autonomous actions which constructively address the challenges posed by the crisis. Thus the adult functions as an "auxiliary ego," a psychological support to affirm and strengthen the child's innate resiliency and adaptability. In this regard, I imagine an adult and child walking together through a heavy spring rainstorm. The adult holds the umbrella, shields the child, guides the way, trusts the child's ability to stay close to avoid the splashes from gutters and puddles, and to match pace with the adult as they go. Yet, the adult also keeps a careful eye on the child's progress, quick to steady the child if he slips from a curb, and be prepared to stop if an ankle turns. Walking through the rainstorm are two vulnerable lives, one more skilled, more prepared to identify and negotiate the hazards, and the other less capable but gaining concrete knowledge of the "how" as the journey with the adult proceeds.

ROLES AND ACTIONS OF HELPING ADULTS

In assisting the child to attain the goal of adaptive coping, the adult often plays several roles, performing in varying ways. Choice of which role or roles as well as how much action is initiated in a particular situation depends primarily on the dynamics inherent in individual circumstances. Nevertheless, this section's identification and discussion of the ways in which an adult can assist children in coping highlights the importance of the adult's words and actions. The adults roles as mediator, information-provider, buffer, provider of coping strategies, referral source, and role model of empowerment are each examined as discrete methods of adult support and assistance.

Adult as Mediator

A central role in most crises situations is the adult's ability to function as a supportive *mediator* of affect and information to the child as he attempts to integrate the critical stress and to formulate adaptive behavior. Within the context of *concerned, caring communicative bonds* already established between adult and child, the adult must *provide honest, age-appropriate, situa-*

tion-specific information. Within the relationship, the adult must have previously communicated an acceptance of the child's affective life, however varied and intense such feelings and expressions may be. In working on the immediate critical issue, the adult must be able to "read" correctly the affects expressed and to respond with empathy and insight. At times this means the adult must sensitively pace provision of information to the child's expressions of understanding and affect. A moving example of this was illustrated recently by Jacobson (1984):

> During a small group time, seven-year-old Beth said, with her thumb in her mouth, "Jeannie, I'm scared." I was surprised and curious, for the story just told was not usually one to elicit fearful responses. "What are you scared of, Beth?" "I'm scared of the bomb." . . . Thus it was that I directly confronted the nuclear issue in the classroom.

Jacobson's trust-filled relationship with her class provided them with a context to express in open discussion the fears, fantasies, and feelings each had about the threat of nuclear destruction. She and her class were then able to discuss, plan, and enact a series of learning activities which affirmed peaceful conflict resolution, thereby beginning the process of turning helpless fright into a sense of empowered social responsibility.

Correctly "hearing" children's affects and ideas often involves an element of interpretative translation whereby the adult communicates not only literal acceptance and comprehension of the child's feelings and thoughts but also verbalizes a sense of *why* those thoughts and ideas are important and *how* they have come to be. In this way, the adult gives credence to the child's current defenses, current ways of coping. Engel (1984) illustrates this point well as she recounts discussion in a 10-year-olds' class on the topic "If I Were Boss of the World." In this nonlinear discussion, children explore the causes and possible solutions to the world's problems. The teacher functions to clarify communication, provide correct information, and to assist in the expression and understanding of affect. It is the teacher, for example, who can attempt to help one child see that his impression that "El Salvador dropped a bomb on American Navy territory" is incorrect, while correctly interpreting his "logic of feeling" which sees events in El Salvador as threatening to American security.

Even more poignant examples of interpretative communication occur in the one-to-one relationships with children in classrooms or therapeutic contexts. McQuade (1985) recounts such a case from her work with a withdrawn 3-year-old girl whose older brother had been severely injured in a fall, resulting in his long-term comatose state. During a play therapy session the child built a tall tower, then seemingly accidentally knocked it over as she moved across the room. She turned pale and said strongly, "I didn't *want* it to fall." The therapist replied quietly, "Nobody *really* wanted Mike to fall." The child studied the therapist's face, then requested to see her mother waiting outside. After a short period of reunion with her mother involving physical contact but no discussion of the incident, the child then returned to the playroom and resumed the building activity. Now, however, the child began to talk about the accident, expressing both her memory of "how and why" as well as her many feelings about what occurred.

Adult as Information-Provider

It cannot be overemphasized that intervention in a crisis situation must be individualized and must occur within the context of a trusting relationship. Explanations, behavioral prescriptions or ready-made solutions cannot be imposed from the outside. Rather, those "on the outside" can caringly extend both emotional support and straightforward, developmentally-geared information which assists the child's intellectual understanding and psychological integration of feelings engendered by this crisis. A recent work by Schwartz and Trabasso (1984) illustrates that children as young as three years can correctly label affect if information and support are consistently supplied by those in their environment. Further, this study finds "children, as well as adults, understand emotions in terms of their antecedent events, concurrent internal states, thoughts and feelings, and consequent actions and expressions" (p. 429). Such capacity makes it incumbent upon adults to find vehicles to assist the growth of understanding about affective states.

Joint reading and discussion of books which either directly delineate or indirectly portray critical issues is often a helpful method. Bernstein's (1979) bibliotherapy compilation is an excellent resource for adults working with children in classrooms or individual sessions. For example, the young boy whose grandfather had died turned repeatedly to two books in play session, one a story about the death of a beloved grandfather and the other about the death of a bird. After several weeks of play sessions, he asked if he could take the books home to "mommy and me-maw" (grandma). Since both these adults expressed their difficulty in talking about the death because they began crying, grieving themselves, I worried about whether they could read and talk with the child. They found, however, that the "stories" made it easier since these served as a vehicle for sharing information and feeling without focusing directly on their loss.

In a similar way, Gardner's (1970, 1983) works are helpful for children whose families are separating or divorcing. In a no-nonsense way he identifies the feelings and conflicts often inherent in family break-ups as well as the possible ways of coping which children can use as their parents establish new life-patterns. As his direct discussions make clear, only when the child can integrate understanding on *cognitive* and *affective* levels will planning for adaptation be possible. Thus, for example, after a child has intellectually and emotionally accepted that his father has abandoned the family, he can spend less time pining for the fantasized father or less time angrily lashing out at "father figures." Rather, he may use the availability of a male relative, teacher, Big Brother, or other community members for support.

Gardner (1977) and many others have also produced parent guidance books for those in search of ways to assist their children in coping effectively. Works by Ramos (1973) and Kuczen (1982) present models of parent guidance which can be utilized by counselors working with children and families. These works are designed to prepare parents for sharing of thought and feeling within the framework of building the child's resilient coping skills.

Yet in using such resources, the caring adult also needs to remember to remain responsive to the child's need to ask, think, integrate, and then ask again as the cyclical linking of information *and* affect slowly coalesce over time. Information imparted once will not easily become part of the child's frame of reference just as directive question-answer sessions will not allow for exploration of feelings and fantasies beyond the "facts." *Sensitive, recurring, open-ended* dialogue is essential. One divorced mother participating in an educator's professional development workshop noted that her adolescent children still would reread *Boy's and Girl's Book About Divorce* (Gardner, 1970), one of the most dog-eared paperbacks in the home, as they become more thoughtful and insightful about the divorce process and single-parent family life-style.

Adult as Buffer

As the adult assists the child in coping, affective expressions of pain, fear or anger may emerge which seem to overwhelm the child. When this occurs, the adult is called upon to provide a containing and strengthening harbor for the sea of emotional tides which are in turmoil. In this sense, the stable adult functions as a *buffer* of stress, helping the child to recognize and understand feelings rather than to simply act them out. Additionally, the caring adult may work to filter stimuli which might trigger emotional upset so that the child's adaptive coping capacities will not be overwhelmed. For example, a preadolescent boy who had been sexually assaulted by another boy and was receiving counseling regarding the incident was urged by his parents to participate in a YMCA summer program. They wanted him to "be one of the boys" again, and they dropped him at the street entrance to the facility. On entering the building, the boy was overcome with panic and spent the day in the family's backyard until the parents returned from work. On learning of the incident, the counselor conferred with the parents about careful planning and facilitating the boy's entrance into programs or activities, since his capacity to handle stress independently was currently limited. After discussion, the parents were able to see that their wish for the boy to "be strong enough" could be accomplished better by actions taken in incremental steps with adults buffering the stressful stimuli inherent in each new situation. Monitoring of media presentations of aggression and sexually was strongly recommended in this case, not to defensively hide such content, but to insure that the boy's growing strengths and skills did not wither under the impact of frightening stimuli.

Adult as Provider of Coping Strategies

Allied with the adult's role as a buffer in the case just described is the adult's role as *provider of coping strategies*. Here the adult might describe a sketch or "groundmap" of alternative actions which can be discussed and evaluated with the child in the safety of the adult-child relationship before actual actions are needed. For the boy in the previous example, for instance, the counselor helped him to distinguish the possible support systems available to him while at home alone, in the neighborhood, community facilities, or in unfamiliar situations. Similarly, a preschool teacher working for the first time with a preschooler whose parents has enacted a joint custody parenting pattern which meant living in two homes on a systematically changing basis described how she prepared the child each Monday for the "schedule of changing homes." Although the signs of stress were often apparent in the child's behavior at preschool by her inability to cope with transition or to initiate active and coherent play with others, the teacher found that preparation and reassurance for all in-school and out-of-school change decreased the child's overt expressions of anxiety and fear. Through words and actions, the teacher clarified her position as helper in providing coping strategies and supports as the child and family established new life patterns.

Adult as Referral Source and Facilitator

However, there will be instances where the types of help, assistance and provision of coping strategies described may prove insufficient. In such cases the helping adult must also function as a *referral source and facilitator* so that the child and/or family can receive professional help and expertise of a more specialized nature. This referral should occur *within the context* of continuing empathic concern for the child. When a child has suffered such a degree of physical or emotional injury that s/he has become withdrawn and isolated, or when the child repetitively plays or describes themes reminiscent of the critical stress in a driven manner, without the growing balance inherent in the healing process, or when the child seems impulsively driven to repeat behaviors that show little connection with immediate social contexts, then individualized professional counseling is absolutely necessary. In such instances, *faith in the health-directed resilient strengths of growing children should not cloud the ability to identify* a child who is developmentally-fixated, and unable to make progress toward adaptation. Growth without intensive assistance from skilled professionals is unlikely, and referral for therapeutic help is a necessity.

Adult as Role Model of Empowered Citizen

Finally, the adult committed to helping children must also dedicate a portion of both professional and personal energies toward the task of creating a safer, more stable and nurturing ecology of childhood. In that capacity, the helping adult provides an active, effective *model of empowerment* to the observing, questing child. Only mature adults are capable of realizing that all life today exists in an interconnected, interdependent macrosystem where trouble and strife in one area of the globe reverberate throughout the communities and countries in the rest of the globe, ringing echoes of anxiety and tension in all individual lives. The truly committed helping adult must form alliances and undertake thoughtful actions to effect long-term conditions of stability and peace. Thus "helpers-of-children" assume responsibility beyond the cradles, classrooms, and communities in their immediate world; they design ways to respond to the hand that reaches out only to find emptiness on the dust of daily bombings or to the drying heat of drought and famine. Creation of the world where growth is not a privilege of the few but an innate right for all young lives, provided by all adults who serve as the guardians and guides of the next generations, is now only a hope, perhaps even only a fantasy. Yet without such a dream the helping adult will only be crisis-responsive, not proactive and future-oriented. With clear articulation such a dream, adults present the child with a model of coherent and committed social activity which attempts to alleviate the conditions of stress and suffering, not just to patch the pieces back together after tragedy. And in this sense the adult's model of being "one who helps to shape the future" strengthens the child's growing sense of entitlement and empowerment, thereby building the capacity to cope creatively and constructively rather than be molded passively by the hands and whims of powerful forces.

SUMMARY

This paper has examined the challenges of contemporary social and global life which are simultaneously presented to growing children and caring adults throughout the world today. After analysis of the multiple domains of critical stress impacting on young lives, discussion of the various roles which the helping adult may enact emphasized the interrelatedness of the primary roles: mediator of affect and information, buffer of stressful stimuli, provider of coping strategies, referral source, and model of empowerment. Through conscious adoption and development of each of these roles, helping adults can work to create more harmonies, stable and growth-producing conditions for children facing the challenges of crisis.

ENDNOTE

1. Judith McQuade is Director of the Child Assessment and Therapy Training program at the Pittsburgh Psychoanalytic Center and has provided verbal communication for clinical examples with this paper.

REFERENCES

Bernstein, J.V. (1979). *Books to help with separation and loss*. New York: Bowker.
Bronfenbrenner, U. (1979). *The ecology of human development: Experiments by nature and design*. Cambridge, MA: Harvard University Press.
Engel, B. (1984). Between feeling and fact: Listening to children. *Harvard Educational Review,* V.54, November 3, 304–314.
Erikson, E. (1950). *Childhood and society*. New York: Norton.
Erikson, E. (1968). *Identity, youth and crisis*. New York: Norton.
Furman, E. (1974). *A child's parent dies: Studies in childhood bereavement*. New Haven: Yale University Press.
Furman. (1978). Helping children cope with death. *Young Children,* 3, 25–32.

Gardner, R. (1970). *Boy's and girl's book about divorce.* New York: Bantam.
Gardner, R. (1977). *The parent's book about divorce,* New York: Bantam.
Gardner, R. (1983). *Boy's and girl's book about one-parent families.* New York: Bantam.
Jacobson, J. (1984). Beginnings. *Harvard Educational Review,* 54, 337–341.
Kliman, G. (1968). *Psychological emergencies of childhood.* New York: Grune & Stratton.
Kliman, G. & Wolfenstein, M. (eds.) (1965). *Children and the death of a president.* New York: Doubleday and Co.
Kuczen, B. (1982). *Childhood Stress: Don't let your child be a victim.* New York: Delacorte Press.
McQuade, Judith. (1985). Personal Communication.
Ramos, S. (1973). *Teaching your child to cope with crisis.* New York: Child Study Press.
Schwartz, R. and Trabasso, T. (1984). Children's understanding of emotions. In Kagan and Zajonc (Eds.), *Emotions, cognition and behavior.* Cambridge: Cambridge University Press.
Terr, L.C. (1979). Children of Chowchilla: A study of psychic trauma. *Psychoanalytic Study of the Child, 34,* 547–623.

The Place of Story in Affective Development: Implications for Educators and Clinicians

Hugh Crago, M Litt, MA

ABSTRACT. The article draws on traditional literary criticism, reader-response research, and the techniques of systemic therapy to synthesize guidelines for teachers and counselors concerned with using story to further the emotional development of children. A theory of reader-story interaction is proposed to explain why some stories are favorites, and the significance of these preferred narratives in an individual's evolving self-concept. Three levels of activity for adult professionals working with children are distinguished. A case is made for individually composed therapeutic stories as an alternative to bibliotherapy.

INTRODUCTION

This article deals with the function of story in the emotional lives of children and with how we as teachers or counselors can best ally ourselves with the therapeutic potential of narrative. Conventionally, in our print-oriented society, we tend to think of stories as synonymous with books, forgetting both oral storytelling and the television set, which is by far the most pervasive source of stories for the majority of children. Because television viewing is considered elsewhere in this volume, I will confine myself mainly to stories read and told. A few references are deliberately retained to TV drama in order to remind us that for many adults and children, story has

---

Hugh Crago is a family therapist in private practice; independent scholar with interests in literature and response to literature, 9 Sullivan Avenue, Wagga Wagga, NSW 2650, Australia.

never had much to do with books and reading. This paper is a personal synthesis of insights gained from three different fields: traditional literary criticism, reader-response research, and systemic family therapy. All are relevant to the part played by story in emotional development, and the best guidelines for teachers and counselors would ideally draw on all three.

TRADITIONAL LITERARY APPROACHES

My original training was in the study of literature in and for itself. As a graduate student in English departments, I learned to suppress many of the thoughts and feelings that came to me as I read a story, and to confine myself to exploring questions like "what makes this book good?" or, "is this book better or worse than others in its genre?" As a reviewer, critic and teacher of literature, I continued for some years to analyze and evaluate books on the basis of my own response to them, but I was uneasily conscious that my neat intellectual structures might have little to do with how individual children, or indeed other adults, thought and felt about those same books. My self-questioning about the validity of the critical approach I had been taught was strengthened by watching my own daughter, Anna, learn the world of story through the picture books we showed and read to her. I assisted my wife, Maureen, in recording five years of interaction between Anna and her books, and there is nothing like record-keeping for forcing yourself to come to terms with facts that do not fit your existing view of the world.

READER-RESPONSE RESEARCH

Our case study (Crago and Crago, 1983) offered evidence of Anna's astonishing capacity to make sense of narratives that some adults might have considered far too complex for her. Anna was not a genius: she did this by organising her understanding of a difficult story around a few concepts that were personally significant to her at a particular age. When, towards the end of our own research, I read Norman Holland's *5 Readers Reading* (1975) the continuity between his work and our own was clear. Holland observed and recorded the spontaneous comments of five college students after reading a short story by Faulkner. He concluded that each student remade the story in his/her own image: each set of comments reflected that reader's personal psychological preoccupations. Not all scholars in the reader-response area would necessarily agree with Holland that texts have no meaning except what the reader projects onto them. More would probably feel comfortable with Rosenblatt's view (1978) that meaning is transacted in a series of ongoing exchanges between reader and text. For applications of response theory to a listening situation rather than a silent reading context, see Crago, 1984; Crago with Travers, 1984. Traditional literary analysis can offer us useful information on how authors achieve *potential effects* through narrative technique, style, and manipulation of viewpoint. But response-research shows that these effects are *only* potential, and subject to massive modification by the receiving apparatus of the individual reader or listener.

The majority of those who write about literature in general, and children's literature in particular, have not yet taken into account the small but highly suggestive body of research findings in reader-response. This renders questionable much run of the mill reviewing of children's books in professional journals. If individual readers or listeners exert so much control over the meaning that a given text will have for them, we cannot claim glibly that a particular book will be enjoyed or rejected by a given age-group, gender-group, or racial group. This is not to say that informed guesses cannot be made on the basis of generalized developmental trends. We cannot, however, know what use an individual will make of a particular story, without precise knowledge of that person in his or her social context. We shall return later to the question of where this leaves "bibliotherapy."

SYSTEMIC FAMILY THERAPY

The literature of developmental psychology has over the past fifty years built up for us a comprehensive map of the stages of normal development for Western children. In particular, those psychologists who have applied and extended Freud's thinking have enabled us to understand and interpret the common signs of emotional disruption in childhood. We can distinguish between predictable and necessary emotional upheavals like adolescent rebellion, and behaviour that signals that the stream of emotional growth has been temporarily dammed or diverted. However, psychology, whether behaviorist or psychoanalytic, has been less than spectacularly successful in its attempts to help emotionally troubled children. In part, this is because affective disturbance has been seen as located within the individual child, rather than within the social system of which that child forms a part. The emerging systemic paradigm, which has given birth to family therapy, steps outside of this limiting view. Just as reader-response research has aided us to consider texts and readers together, as an interactive system, so family therapy invites us to consider "problem behavior" as meaningful and functional within a wider social context. Not only has family therapy conceptualized emotional illness differently from traditional psychology, it has also popularised new techniques for intervention in troubled families, especially in its use of *therapeutic story*. Family therapy has connected with my earlier interest in literature in unexpected and exciting ways.

STORY IN AFFECTIVE DEVELOPMENT

The Universality of Story

Stories are part of almost every human's life from a very early age, whether in the form of parental anecdote, television cartoon, or picture-book. Hearing or seeing stories provides young children with models of how experience can be shaped and organised into meaningful patterns. It is a rare preschooler who does not imitate the models that are available to her by creating stories of her own. These may be monologues that are spoken aloud with or without an audience (Crago and Crago, 1983; Evans, 1983; Fox, 1983), narrative commentary muttered while playing, or pictures drawn with or without verbal accompaniment. Sutton-Smith and his co-workers have shown that this "storying" is not confined to children from middle-class or professional backgrounds (1980). If story is part of children's environment, it cannot fail to play a part in their affective development. Adult-created stories offer events, characters and feelings with which children may identify; child-created stories function as an emotional laboratory, in which they can express, manipulate and gain perspective on their own feelings. Of the multitude of adult-told stories in a child's early experience, though, some will have little impact, while others will make a deep and lasting impression. A six year old girl wants to hear the tale of "Cinderella" over and over again. An eleven year old boy watches "Knight Rider" religiously every week. Why are these stories so important, and not others?

The Roots of Preference

At any given stage of development, for a given child, particular stories will seem special because they embody themes which are both appropriate to that child's developmental phase, and to the specific features of that child's personality. It is *not* a matter of *literal* similarities between the content of a story and the surface details of a child's own life. The girl who requests "Cinderella" again and again is not a scorned step-sister, nor in a more general sense a physically neglected child. The eleven year old fan of Michael Knight is a boy of below-average intelligence whose parents own a very ordinary automobile. Rather, stories are selected by children as "special" on the basis of metaphoric, or symbolic correspondence to the child's interior construction of reality. The shape of the story needs to parallel the shape the child has unconsciously given to his or her experiences. A child from a materially comfortable home, with a reasonably caring family, may still feel inside like a left-out, put-down Cinderella. A boy may not own a magic car like KIT in "Knight Rider", but he does have a mother who is intelligent, purposeful and mindful of his welfare in the same way that KIT takes care of Michael Knight. In their chosen stories, there may be much that is alien or irrelevant to this boy and girl. That does not matter, because the story still holds a power and a meaning for them on the basis of the elements they have unconsciously selected from it, elements which metaphorically reflect their own experience. Neither child would, if you asked, be able to tell you why the chosen story was so significant to them, and both would almost certainly reject the explanation just offered. All that means is that the transaction they are making with the texts is an unconscious one, and all the more powerful for that.

Is Quality Relevant?

The concerns and techniques of literary criticism are not of much value in determining why particular stories appeal so strongly to individuals. Genre distinctions are certainly irrelevant. It is not important whether a given story is "fantasy" or "realism", whether it is "contemporary" or "historical". When questioned, a child may say that she likes "stories about the past" or "mysteries" but it will often transpire, when you know the child's reading history better, that she actually means "I like stories that remind me of *X*", where "X" was a story that metaphorically fitted the child's inner experience, and *happened* to belong to the historical or mystery genre. The only funtional significance in fantasy/realism or familiar/exotic distinctions is that many children, and adults too, seem to need the distancing effect provided by a narrative set in another world, or in a faroff time or place, in order to accept the metaphoric parallel that it offers to their own experience. The distancing effect will be especially important when we come to discuss the composing of therapeutic stories in the *Recommendations* section below.

Similarly, the issue of literary quality rarely arises in the context of children's personal choices. Trained critics focus on aspects of narrative art like credible dialogue, rounded characterisation, convincing plot-structure and fresh, original language, but at the level of unconscious emotional investment in a particular tale, such things simply do not matter. Indeed, it could be argued with some plausibility that many children and adults find it easier to pour their psychic contents into vessels that are relatively featureless. Solid, individualistic characters may be harder to identify with than superheroes with just a few stereotyped traits. The protagonists of "series" fiction and television are like this, and unlike a single novel, series books and TV shows offer the potent appeal of endless repetition of the same formula. Language that is precise and vivid demands a degree of submission to a range of meanings controlled by the author. Language that is generalized and full of clichés can more readily be filled with the reader's own personal meanings. Literary quality has little to do with the process by which children make certain stories their own, but it does have a place for teachers and librarians who want to extend children's options. This is discussed further in *Recommendations*.

How Story Choices Influence Affective Development

My sense of the way story and personality interact in individuals is summed up in the phrase "stories make us make stories" (Crago, unpublished, 1985). As already stated, we select narratives because of their correspondence with our inner lives. Those stories then offer a specific shape and a range of images that focus and refine our existing self-pictures, and encourage us to become more fully and intensely what we already are. An emotionally healthy person will be able to seek out stories that extend, as well as confirm, his or her self-image. The less emotionally healthy we are the less we would be able to cope with any stories but those which simply confirm. Out of our newly-focussed selves, we then search for more stories that resemble the originally formative ones, and we may also begin to create within our heads, or in writing, stories of our own that express the formative elements that first attracted us.

As a boy of about seven, I read Hans Christian Andersen's "The Snow Queen", and it became my favorite among his tales. I was an introverted, shy child, sensitive to real or imagined slights from others. I *was* little Kay, the story's hero. For me the tale's most compelling image was the description of Kay alone on the frozen lake in the Snow Queen's palace, fruitlessly trying to arrange the pieces of ice so that they would form the word "Eternity". I could not have explained then what this meant to me. But as I grew up, I did exactly what Kay did in the story: I retreated from people who might hurt or reject me into a life of puzzle-solving in the palace of my mind. It was not until I had reached my early thirties, and emotions were reasserting themselves in my life, that I recalled the Andersen tale, and realised how I had used it to form an extreme and unncessarily dramatic concept of my self. Only as I write this do I realise something else. In the story, Kay was redeemed by Gerda's love, and returns to normal life. What might my own life have been like if Kay had stayed in the Snow Queen's palace forever?

Interestingly enough, it was also around the age of thirty that I became engrossed in Hesse's adult novel, *The Glass Bead Game.* More aware of my inner life than I had been at seven, I quickly saw why this story was so important to me. Once again, I had selected a story that presented me with the seductive image of a self-contained life of pure intellect. It way Kay in the ice palace all over again. But this time there was a significant difference. Unlike Kay, Hesse's hero himself perceives the limitations of his chosen life-course, takes responsibilty for himself, and eventually returns to the world. Being personally in a stage of life-transition, I was able to use the novel as a model in a conscious way, to aid me in my own journey. *The Glass Bead Game* was not only more developmentally appropriate to me at thirty: it was also therapeutic.

Developmental Functions of Story-types

This issue of the match between particular types of stories and given developmental stages has recently been explored by a number of writers. Less pretentious and more convincing than Bettelheim's (1976) better-known analysis, is the work of Favat (1977) who lays out the detailed correspondences between fairytale discourse and the thinking processes of young children, thereby offering a better explanation than we have hitherto had of the enduring popularity of folk literature among them. Favat can be read in conjunction with Nodelman's (1977) essay, one of the rare literary analyses that offers insights into the function and appeal of stories. Nodelman also explores the appeal of the super-hero (1983) and Schlager (1978) provides a brief but useful account of the ways that particular children's classics match or fail to match the developmental concerns of middle childhood. The teacher who has been puzzled by the fact that some "quality" texts are consistently popular with her classes while others fail to excite any interest at all will find these references enlightening.

Our new awareness of the usefulness of matching stories with developmental stages should not lead us to forget that there are times when stories offer vicarious experience of feelings and situations well in *advance* of a child's chronological age. In other words, a story may provide a child with a sort of advance map of a particular feeling-territory. The obvious example is love and sexuality. Latency-age girls do not read Judy Blume's *Forever* (1975) simply because it deals with sex explicitly and is disapproved of by some adults. They read and re-read it because it tells them in *narrative* form "what it's going to feel like"—something no factual sex manual can tell them. My daughter read *Forever* several times, beginning at about age ten. She had no boyfriend, and was not seeking a mirroring of her current "public" life. Nor was she seeking a deep, symbolic correspondence with her inner life. She simply wanted a chance to live for a few hours in her own possible future, to leap into early adulthood for awhile in complete safety. When she actually reaches that stage in her life, the story, dimly-recalled or totally forgotten, may well have provided her with advance information about the new experiences she will be encountering.

RECOMMENDATIONS

In this section I shall distinguish three levels at which an adult professional may operate when conscious of the importance of story in the emotional growth of children:

1. the level of *response* to the child's independent story-choices and story-making.
2. the level of *reader-guidance or conferencing,* where the adult will seek to broaden or deepen the artistic experience the child is independently creating or seeking out.
3. the level of *conscious therapeutic intervention* when a child's normal emotional growth has been blocked.

Obviously, in practice the levels cannot always be neatly demarcated, and there will be exceptions to the categories I have suggested. Like all formulas, mine should be regarded critically, rather than followed slavishly. Hopefully, these categories will introduce greater clarity into what has become a rather confused, if well-meaning, set of precepts and practices.

The Level of Response

At this level, the professional needs to know how to accept in an open-minded, supportive way whatever a child may offer in the way of comment on stories he has read or heard. This is not as easy as it sounds, especially for teachers used to commenting critically on almost everything a child says, or for those who themselves have strong opinions about the value or worthlessness of certain stories. However, it is a *sine qua non* if children are to feel safe to express and explore their responses to stories. The teacher or librarian allows children to select stories freely. She does not ask "why" questions, which block the child's spontaneity, and rarely produce the kinds of insight that the professional is presumably hoping for. In our own work with Anna in her preschool years, we found that the best way to encourage her to talk about a story was to ask no questions at all, but instead to venture an opinion of our own, especially if it restated or built upon something she had already said about the tale in question. The aim was not to be an equal partner in the conversation, but simply to model for Anna the kind of uncensored, transparent statement we hoped she would make. In assisting older children to explore their response to a narrative, open-ended questions are more productive than ones that expect a pre-determined answer, and a climate of informality seems to aid children to venture a wide range of perceptions, questions and speculations (Crago, 1982). When it is children's own compositions that are in question, the same guidelines apply. "Tell me some more about . . . " or "I really liked the bit where you made him say . . . " are going to get you further than responses like "why did you say . . . " or "why don't you . . . "

The Level of Reader-Guidance

At this level, the professional plays a more obviously active part than at the level of response, but still needs to be more empathic and supportive than I suspect many classroom teachers manage to be. In discussing how teachers should offer feedback to students on their own pieces of writing. Graves (1978) and Clifford (1981) describe the writing "conference", in which the teacher responds in a way that helps a child to realize more of the potential of his piece, without actually telling him what to write or how to express his thoughts. Similar principles apply when we are dealing with children's choices from among adult-composed stories. A teacher or librarian who is able to function well at the *response* level will already possess some knowledge of a particular child's pattern of story-choices. She will know something of the kinds of themes that fire him, and the kind of style he likes. She will have noted the stories to which he returns a second and a third time, read or listened to these stories herself, and begun to form a hypothesis about what draws him to them. She will have registered any similarities between his favorites.

With this awareness, the professional can begin cautiously to recommend stories that may broaden or deepen the literary or visual treatment of the child's preferred themes. Here traditional literary values again become relevant, for the author of a critically-approved story may have conveyed the emotional life of her characters more specifically and more accurately than the author of a pot-boiler. If the pot-boiler is the child's first, spontaneous favorite, then care must be taken to select the correct recommendation—one which carries the same themes, and offers the reader enhanced understanding of those themes, without being so demanding linguistically or structurally that it is simply rejected as "too hard".

If this sounds too delicate and difficult to be possible, help is at hand in two forms. The first is the well-known fact that film, audiotape and (especially) expert reading aloud are all ways of bridging the gap between a demanding text and a child reader who may be ready for its theme, but ill-prepared for its literary complexity. We are all aware of how children will avidly read a novel if they have first been impressed by a filmed version, and of how a good oral reader can make even a sophisticated, adult-level narrative comprehensible and interesting for an audience far younger than its author originally intended. The second is the realization that sometimes a story that will take a reader further into emotional awareness of his preferred theme may be one that is officially written for an audience *younger* than he is. William Armstrong's *Sounder* 1969) proved to be a far better introduction for an eighteen-year old college student of mine to literary treatments of oppression than any number of adult novels would have been: his skills for reading sophisticated texts were undeveloped at that point. Similarly, Elaine Moss (1978) points out that complex, sophisticated picture books are often more appropriately recommended to older Elementary or even Junior High School age groups than to the young children for whom they were ostensibly published.

The Level of Conscious Therapeutic Intervention

At the first and second levels, the adult professional is relying on a child's innate sense of what she needs at a particular developmental stage, trying to enrich, perhaps, but not to alter fundamentally the experiences the child is voluntarily seeking out. In the third level, the professional is aware of a block in the child's normal emotional development, and wants to use the therapeutic power of narrative to help dissolve this block. Hence caution and special skills are called for. Traditionally, "bibliotherapy" has meant that a librarian, teacher or counselor, recommends a particular story to a child with a problem because its hero has a problem similar to the child's, but is able to resolve it. There are two big difficulties with this. First, the chosen story is unlikely to match the child's situation exactly, and may differ considerably in some aspects. In itself, at a literal level, that might not matter. Many children would *reject* a story that too obviously duplicates their situation, and too transparently offers them a solution to their problems. But if the recommended narrative does not correspond at a deep level with the child's inner reality, then it is unlikely to be therapeutic at all.

The issue then becomes how to find a story that possesses this symbolic correspondence, and yet which is not, in its literal content, too obviously close to the details of the child's own life. This demands extensive knowledge both of the child, and of the world of children's literature.

Here we encounter a second difficulty. A child's problem, if it is serious enough to need professional intervention, is unlikely to be "in" the child himself: it is part of a wider context, part of a pattern of feelings and interactions in his family, his peer group or his classroom. A therapeutic story that fails to take this into account, and simply shows a hero resolving a problem without concommitant changes in his context, is unlikely to be very helpful, though it may do no harm.

The best therapeutic stories are written especially for individual children by their counselor. Obviously, this refers to short stories, not whole novels. Gordon (1978) explains in detail how such stories can embody the necessary parallels between the client's own life situation and the structure of the narrative, but can be devised so that there is no literal or surface resemblance between the setting and characters of the story and the client's world. Specially-written therapeutic stories can have built into them an understanding of the way the child's problem is related to, and kept active by, the behavior of significant others in this world. Operating through metaphor, the story may have the power to bypass consciousness. Suggested solutions that it contains may be accepted by the child and his family, where those same suggestions would almost certainly be rejected if offered as direct advice in a face to face counseling session, or if offered in the form of a story that literally paralleled the child's situation. Park (1982) describes a technique whereby the therapist drafts her story, then reads it aloud to the child, asking him to fill in key words that tell how the protagonist would think and feel. The child thus becomes co-composer, and "owns" the story more fully—but within a structure controlled by the therapist. Parents can read therapeutic stories to children at bedtime, and can themselves be addressed by the stories, indirectly, and in humane and face-saving ways. Older children can be given their personal copy of the story and asked to illustrate it.

I have myself just composed a 1000-word story for the young fan of "Knight Rider" whom we met earlier in this paper. It is called "The Inside Story of Michael Knight" and in it the wonder-car, KIT, plays the same role for the hero as my young client's mother plays in his life. Eleven year old Scott is unlikely ever to perceive that the story metaphorically describes him and his family, but he will find in it some suggestions that may help him resolve a longstanding speech inhibition. His mother, who will read the story with him, may also gain some new insight into his problem. I should emphasize that I know his mother well, and have worked with her in therapy before. Therapeutic story is not a "quickie" intervention, nor a panacaea for all sorts of crisis. It does however offer an elegant, indirect way of helping children and their families out of impasses, and demonstrates the power of story to alter the course of lives, instead of merely confirming it.

REFERENCES

Bettelheim, B. (1976). *The uses of enchantment.* New York: Knopf.

Clifford, J. (1981). Composing in stages: The effects of collaborative pedagogy. *Research in the Teaching of English, 15* (1).

Crago, H. (1982). "I like a REAL story": A case study of literary response at age nine. *Developments in English Teaching* (Australia), *1* (3).

Crago, H. (1984). "Once upon a time there was—Wendy! Sit down!" *Orana* (Australia), *20* (1).

Crago, H. with Travers, M. (1984). The opening door: Reader, text and child listeners as a novel begins. *Developments in English Teaching* (Australia), *3* (1).

Crago, H. (1985). *Stories make us make stories.* Unpublished manuscript.

Crago, M., & Crago, H. (1983). *Prelude to literacy.* Carbondale, IL: Southern Illinois, University Press.

Evans, W.D. (1983). Telling first stories. *Developments in English Teaching* (Australia), *2* (3).

Favat, A. (1977). *Child and tale: The origins of interest.* Urbana, IL: National Council of Teachers of English.

Fox, C. (1983). Talking like a book: Young children's oral monologues. In M. Meek (Ed.), *Opening moves. Bedford way papers 17.* London: University of London Institute of Education.

Gordon, D. (1978). *Therapeutic metaphors.* Cupertino, CA: Meta Publications.

Graves, D. (1978). Research update. We won't let them write. *Language Arts,* 635–640.

Holland, N. (1975). *5 readers reading.* New Haven: Yale University Press.

Moss, E. (1978). Them's for the infants, Miss: Some misguided attitudes to picture books for the older reader. *Signal, 26, 27.*

Nodelman, P. (1977). What makes a fairy tale good: The queer kindness of "The Golden Bird". *Children's Literature in Education, 26* (Autumn).

Nodelman, P. (1983, May). Some heroes have freckles. *Children and their literature: A reading book.* Lafayette, IN: Children's Literature Association Publications.

Park, S. (1982). The dog and the crocodile: The use of story writing in the therapy of families with young children. *Australian Journal of Family Therapy, 4* (1).

Rosenblatt, L. (1978). *The reader, the text, the poem.* Carbondale, ILL: Southern Illinois University Press.

Schlager, N. (1978). Predicting children's choices in literature: A developmental approach. *Children's Literature in Education,* 30 (Autumn).

Sutton-Smith, B., Abrams, D.M., Botvin, G. J., Caring, M.L., Gildesgame, D. P., Mahony, H.H., & Stevens, T. R. (1980). *The folkstories of children.* Philadelphia: University of Pennsylvania Press.

Summary

Sally Provence, MD

This volume attests to the sophistication of the participating authors about the importance of emotions in the development of the child and their concern about the relative neglect of emotions as a focus of child development research. It is not possible to summarize a volume such as this, even though there is the unifying theme of children's feelings. Each paper deserves reading in its entirety. Some are of greatest interest to those involved in teaching or clinical practice. Others are particularly helpful in the presentation and discussion of research issues. The choice of topics and ideas covered in this essay, then, is admittedly selective and cannot do justice to the whole.

Michael Lewis' article "The Role of Emotion in Development" is persuasive in its informed and sophisticated discussion of relationships between emotions and the individual's course of life. He reminds us for example that emotional and motor cues were used by Piaget and many other investigators to assess cognitive abilities in young children. He charts a path for future studies and cautions us about the disadvantages of neglecting emotions in our efforts to understand development more clearly. Lewis has been one of the few investigators who has seen the need and addressed it in his studies.

Few would challenge the idea that feelings are continuous aspects of our lives and that they are basic to the social relatedness of the human family. The preadaptedness of the human infant, and his readiness at birth for social interaction has become generally acknowledged. The importance of affects in social signalling at early ages, and especially in the interactions between infant and caregiver can hardly be over-

---

Sally Provence is Professor of Pediatrics, Yale Child Study Center, P.O. Box 3333, New Haven, CT 06510.

emphasized. These insights, however, are fairly recent. The relative neglect of theoretical advances in respect to affects occurred, curiously enough, in psychoanalysis as well as in other psychologies. Jacobson (1954), in pointing out that Freud's first theory of neurosis was an affect theory, suggested that the development of instinct theory greatly delayed efforts to advance and clarify the concept of affects and their relationship to other aspects of development.

Among the new generation of psychoanalyst investigators, the work of Greenspan (1981), Emde (1980), Emde et al. (1976), Sander (1964, 1975, 1980), Shapiro and Stern (1980) and Stern (1974) reflects the renewed interest in the systematic study of the emotions.

Emde's (1980) article summarizes a number of attitudes, based on research and clinical practice, that are particularly relevant as guides to current thinking and study: the infant is fundamentally active and preadapted to seek social contact and other stimuli; he is involved in transactions with others from the beginning onward; affects exist as primary (psychobiological) structures early in development; and are seen as adaptive and as organizing influences on activity, thought, defense and symptoms; emotions are inseparable from cognition.

Stanley Greenspan's introduction to this volume makes similar points. Lewis and Strayer in their essays have pulled together much of the research on affect that informs us about what is currently being done to study them. The availability of technologies not available 20 years ago is one of the new steps. But there is also a new way of thinking about new and old observations that is linked especially to the adaptive nature of emotions and their vital importance in social interaction.

The paper of Piers and Curry contains, among other valuable comments, the statement that "The organizing and propelling force of affects enhance, enliven or retard and stultify development at all ages. Their utilization of Erikson's psychosocial theory to provide a framework for looking at infants, toddlers, preschool and school age children is followed by sensitive and sound suggestions for parents and teachers.

Curry's concern about young children who do not play and teachers who do not value play as significant for the child's emotional *and* cognitive development strikes a responsive chord in all who are persuaded of their inseparability. It reminds us anew that out understanding of children and our effectiveness as educators and clinicians is hampered by the neglect of feelings in the life of the child. The extent to which cognitive measures have come to determine much of social policy for children is, as Lewis says, a disturbing state in need of correction.

Gilbert Foley's presentation of a newly developed Attachment-Separation-Individuation Scale grew out of interest in determining whether aspects of Mahler's (1975) theories regarding separation and individuation in the life of the infant, could be operationalized for investigators and practitioners. While the method of observation and scales for mother and infant were initially developed to permit a more clear understanding of the psychological development of the handicapped child, it seems very likely that they will be very useful for other groups of infants and toddlers also.

The paper of Jerome and Dorothy Singer on television viewing and family communication styles as predictions of children's emotional behavior presents aspects of their ongoing studies on the influence of television. An important focus of this paper is on the significance of the parent mediation, or the lack of it, on how affective and cognition growth of preschool and school-age children will be influenced. The paper is a very instructive discussion of some of the more important issues. Links between imaginative play and feelings, for example, are among the topics examined. The significance of the interaction between family patterns including whether parents actively mediate the outside world including the world of television is persuasively elucidated.

Crago's essay on the place of the story in affective development points out from another perspective how a child perceives and makes use of material in accordance with what is significant in his or her life at the time. Crago introduces ideas that are compatible with others who emphasize phase-specific developmental trends, and also point out that individual features of a child's personality will influence how the story is experienced and used. His discussion of the therapeutic use of the personal story is usually superior to one chosen from a book is convincing and congenial with what therapists of young children would expect.

Dimidjian's discussion of the importance of adults in helping children in times of crisis and how their role can be conceptualized spells out some of the ways in which adults, whether teacher, parents or others, can enable children to deal with stress. The importance of the sensitivity of the adult to an individual child in appreciating the child's feelings as well as the role of familitator of the child's developing ability to face challenges is convincing. The role is especially difficult when stress is chronic and punctuated by recurrent crisis as in the case in many families.

Finally, the information, experience and concern for children expressed in this timely volume by sophisticated and dedicated practitioners and investigators should lend support for a greater commitment to the consideration of children's feelings.

REFERENCES

Emde, R.N. (1980). Toward a psychoanalytic theory of affect I and II. In S. I. Greenspan & G. H. Pollock (Eds.), *The course of life: Psychoanalytic contributions toward understanding personality development: Vol. 1. Infancy and early childhood* (pp. 63–112, DHHS Publication No. ADM 80-786). Washington, DC: U.S. Government Printing Office.

Emde, R. N., Gaensbauer, T.J., & Harmon, R. J. (1976). *Emotional expression in infancy: A biobehavioral study. Psychological Issues. Monograph 37.* New York: International Universities Press.

Greenspan, S. I. (1981). *Psychopathology and adaptation in infancy and early childhood: Principles of clinical diagnosis and preventive intervention.* New York: International Universities Press.

Jacobson, E. (1954). The sex and the object world. *Psychoanalytic Study of the Child, 9,* 75–87.

Mahler, M. S., Pine, F. & Bergman, A. (1975). *The psychological birth of the human infant.* New York: Basic Books.

Sander, L. W. (1964). Adaptive relationships in early mother-child interaction. *Journal of the Academy of Child Psychiatry, 3*(2), 231–264.

Sander, L. W. (1975). Infant and caretaking environment: Investigation and conceptualization of adaptive behavior in a system of increasing complexity. In E. J. Anthony (Ed.), *Explorations in child psychiatry* (pp. 129–166). New York: Plenum Press.

Sander, L. W. (1980). Investigation of the infant and its caretaking environment as a biological system. In S.I. Greenspan & G. H. Pollock (Eds.), *The course of life: Psychoanalytic contributions toward understanding personality development: Vol. 1. Infancy and early childhood* (pp. 117–202, DHHS Publication No. ADM 80–786). Washington, DC: U.S. Government Printing Office.

Shapiro, T., & Stern, D. (1980). Psychoanalytic perspectives on the first year of life–The establishment of the object in an affective field. In S. I. Greenspan & G. H. Pollock (Eds.), *The course of life: Psychoanalytic contributions toward under-*

standing personality development: Vol. I. Infancy and early childhood (pp. 113–128, DHHS Publication No. ADM 80-786). Washington, DC: U.S. Government Printing Office.

Stern, D. (1974). Mother and infant at play: The dyadic interaction involving facial, vocal and gaze behavior. In M. Lewis & L. Rosenblum (Eds.), *The effect of the infant on its caregiver.* New York: John Wiley and Sons.

SELECTED READINGS

ERIC Documents and Journal Articles

ERIC DOCUMENTS

BIBLIOTHERAPY. FACT SHEET. ERIC Clearinghouse on Reading and Communication Skills. (1982)

Defines bibliotherapy and discusses who should conduct it, when and how it can be used, and limitations of the approach. Includes lists of techniques for accurately determining the needs of students, basic procedures in conducting bibliotherapy, and resources. (ED 234 338; 4p.)

CHILDREN'S UNDERSTANDING OF FEELINGS: A MATTER OF POINT OF VIEW. Ellen D. Nannis and Philip A. Cowan. (1983)

Investigates how first-, third-, and fifth-grade children understand feelings in themselves and their parents. Composite scores were created by averaging scores on questions involving one, two, and three points of view. Tests indicated that answers invoking a single point of view invoked more sophisticated criteria than did answers involving two or three points of view. (ED 238 582; 16p.)

HOW TO GENERATE VALUES IN YOUNG CHILDREN: INTEGRITY, HONESTY, INDIVIDUALITY, SELF-CONFIDENCE, AND WISDOM. Sue Spayth Riley. (1984)

Provides an early childhood educator's anecdotal experiences and insights and emphasizes the importance of developing decision-making capabilities in young children. Argues that children should be given freedom to learn from their own experiences and from the consequences of their actions. (ED 247 019; 103p.)

LEARNING THROUGH IMPROVISATIONAL GAMES. Scottie Putman. (1983)

Describes the usefulness of improvisational gaming, a technique that makes use of intuition, sense-memory, and imagination to teach social skills as well as subject matter. Points out the importance of objective and nonjudgmental feedback to a successful process. (ED 237 161; 4p.)

FILMS AND FEELINGS. Maureen Gaffney, Ed. (1981)

Collects articles focusing on children's emotional responses to films. The first article describes a methodology and rationale for using story films to encourage children's exploration of their feelings; the second illustrates specific techniques for using films with children; the third concerns the use of media as a means for bringing feelings into the classroom; and the fourth provides reviews of seven films. (ED 241 006; 21p.)

TELL ME HOW YOU FEEL . . . CREATING AN AWARENESS OF EMOTIONS IN A DAY CARE SETTING. Cathy Schmidt and Helen M. Harvey. (1981)

Describes four experiences designed to increase adult awareness of the child's perspective in adult-child dyadic interaction and outlines 12 children's activities to encourage concentration on feelings in a positive group situation. (ED 245 810; 17p.)

JOURNAL ARTICLES

INSTRUCTIONAL THEORIES: MAXIMIZING THEIR STRENGTHS FOR APPLICATION. Barbara L. Martin and Marcy P. Driscoll. *Performance and Instruction,* 1984, 23(6), 1–4.

Briefly explores the philosophical underpinnings and points of view of several instructional theories: behavioral, cognitive information processing, cognitive inquiry, and humanism. Examines goals, instructional processes, and evaluation strategies for each orientation.

THE LANGUAGE OF FEELINGS: A PROGRAM IN AFFECTIVE EDUCATION. Jackson Taylor. *Momentum,* 1984, 15(1), 47–49.

Offers seven lesson plans to help blend the affective and cognitive realms of children's learning. Plans connect an emotional lexicon with written and spoken dialogues, photographs, arguments, and movements.

SHARING IS . . . VIEWS FROM 3-YEAR-OLDS AND THOUGHTS FOR TEACHERS. Stevie Hoffman and Becky Wundram. *Childhood Education,* 1984, 60(4), 261–65.

Discusses how children learn to share, gives three examples of children's sharing behavior, and raises issues concerning the teaching of sharing skills.

THE ROLE OF COGNITIVE DEVELOPMENT IN CHILDREN'S UNDERSTANDINGS OF THEIR OWN FEELINGS. Jacqueline J. Carroll and Margaret S. Steward. *Child Development,* 1984, 55(4), 1486–92.

Investigates the relationship between cognitive and affective processes in 4- and 5-year olds. Children were interviewed individually, administered a series of Piagetian tasks, and given the Peabody Picture Vocabulary Test. Affective and cognitive performance were found to be significantly correlated.

WHAT CAN SCHOOLS BECOME? Selma Wasermann. *Phi Delta Kappan,* 1984, 65(10), 688–89.

Points out that the increase in computer-assisted learning demands that schools reassess their reasons for being and emphasize the nurturing of children's feelings; the promotion of interpersonal and higher-level cognitive skills; and the development of creativity, imagination, and moral integrity.

ABOUT ERIC

ERIC, the Educational Resources Information Center, is funded by the National Institute of Education. Included in the ERIC system are 16 separate clearinghouses, each responsible for collecting and disseminating information on a specific subject area in education. The ERIC Clearinghouse on Elementary and Early Childhood Education (ERIC/EECE) deals with information relating to the education and development of children from birth through age 12.

ERIC DOCUMENTS are cited and abstracted in the monthly index *Resources in Education (RIE).* Most ERIC documents may be read on microfiche in libraries and information centers. In addition, the majority can be ordered in paper copy and/or on microfiche from the ERIC Document Reproduction Service, PO Box 190, Arlington, VA 22210. For complete information on how to order, contact EDRS or consult the most recent issue of *RIE.*

JOURNAL ARTICLES are cited and annotated in the monthly publication *Current Index to Journals in Education (CIJE);* journals may be read at libraries or ordered through subscription. Selected article reprints are available from University Microfilms International, Article Reprint Department, 300 N. Zeeb Road, Ann Arbor, MI 48106. Please see the most recent issue of *CIJE* for UMI ordering details.

Further information about the ERIC network and services of ERIC/EECE is available from ERIC/EECE Information Services, College of Education, University of Illinois, 805 W. Pennsylvania Ave., Urbana, IL 61801. Telephone (217) 333-1386.

Index

